Angelique + Aida

Nature Cure

A Guide to Healthy Living

Nature Cure

A Guide to Healthy Living

BELINDA GRANT VIAGAS
ND, DO, DipC

Newleaf

Newleaf

an imprint of
Gill & Macmillan Ltd
Goldenbridge
Dublin 8
with associated companies throughout the world
www.gillmacmillan.ie

0 7171 2773 7
Print origination by Carole Lynch
Printed by The Guernsey Press

This book is typeset in 11/14 pt Bembo

A CIP catalogue record for this book is available from the British Library.

1 3 5 4 2

DEDICATION

To Nora, my mother,
who has shared her love of the natural world with me
for as long as I can remember

CONTENTS

ACKNOWLEDGMENTS

Judy Love blessed me with her kindness and friendship, and enabled this book in so many ways. I cherish the memories of the late Paola Toso, 'my beautifull sister', and I give thanks for knowing my late father, Henry Anthony Viagas. Bridget Brown always pointed me in the right direction, and my world would not be complete without O'Connors and the joys of the Friday morning gang. I appreciate my friends and allies who gave their love, support, and valuable teachings, and treasure the gift of my beloved storyteller and special friend.

Chapter 1

INTRODUCTION

Nature offers us an abundant richness of methods, techniques, exercises, remedies and cures. They are all simple, safe and effective, and work to support and enhance our own health. They are as old as the planet, and have carried humankind this far, keeping people well and sustaining us through all we have encountered. Many of these simple, natural ways are steeped in ancient lore, but have been forgotten or disregarded in the last generation or so. This is the Natural Wisdom of our forbears, the green witchcraft of midwives and Wise Women and Shamans throughout the centuries, and it is just as powerful and relevant to life today as it ever was.

Nature Cure embraces a wide range of skills and techniques, and draws on a variety of natural and readily available resources to allow us an immediate and easy-to-use form of healthcare.

The wonder of Nature Cure is that it embraces so many different ways that all work together in harmony to support the balance, full health and happiness of every one of us. These different aspects of healing work with the many strands of our experience, from our emotional well-being to the reality of our physical form, from the sacred to the material, and from the everyday to the special. They all share a fundamental truth: that we are not separate from the natural world, and that this is where the storehouse of our health and energy is based. We can experience the truth of this for ourselves every day. Simply opening the curtains in the morning and looking out at the weather can place our perceptions and feelings about ourselves in a much wider context. Spending time outdoors in the natural world can have a profoundly beneficial effect upon our entire organism, balancing and revitalising us. Bringing nature indoors through using the fruits of the earth and the elements of life, connects us in a very real way with the whole of creation. It also makes available to us a simple and direct method for healing our own ills.

Eating well, using food as medicine, respecting the body's needs and finding the most straightforward ways to honour them puts us at the centre of a powerful system of cure that is elegant in its simplicity. Nature Cure is about the wealth of ways that we may support the body in its own best efforts, and gently encourage it to respond, enhancing its own drive towards full health. Nature Cure embraces all those ways of working with the whole person that will not interfere with or intrude upon the subtle integrity of the system. This includes those techniques such as meditation or personal reflection that encourage us to find peace and to know ourselves better, as well as practical skills such as self-diagnosis and hydrotherapy. It means using every natural means at our disposal, and uncovering our own reservoir of health-giving energy and inspiration. It is about uncapping the resources that are within and around us, and allowing them to carry us forward on a tide of good health. Fundamentally, Nature Cure is about understanding ourselves and our place in the world. It is about discovering how to maximise our individual constitutional strengths and harness our inherent ability to right any imbalances. It is about believing in ourselves and in our own capacity for maximum health and happiness.

Optimum health and vitality, ample energy and a sense of well-being are the most natural, normal things in the world for every one of us to enjoy. Natural healthcare is about enabling that in a very active way — supporting, enhancing, encouraging and fostering a way to maximise our own personalised and unique recipe for full health.

The sum total of our experience governs our health. It is maintained as a delicate balance that requires only a light touch to tip the scales. Nature Cure is about learning to use a feather-like touch in order to meet this subtle, shifting energy and make it smile.

The world is made from the same raw material as ourselves. The body comprises the same elements that we see around us and that constitute our earthly home and its environment. Naturally, it makes total sense that we should respond most fully and easily to an aspect of nature, allowing it to resonate with something within ourselves and thereby heal us. Keeping our lives simple and straightforward means maintaining full health in the easiest of ways. Using natural methods to reinforce our health and well-being reduces the need to resort to synthetic palliatives and pharmaceutical drugs. On a biochemical level the chemicals and substitutes that we eat and use most frequently can cause terrible confusion, leading to allergic responses and difficulties with absorption and the availability of physical energy. When the body is faced with a compound that it does not recognise, enormous amounts of energy become tied up in endeavouring to deal with it. This is what happens every time we breathe air that is not clean and eat food that has been chemically grown and treated, synthesised and processed, or genetically altered.

Pharmaceutical drugs tend to act like a knock-out punch — flooding the body with a synthetic chemical in extreme doses, far beyond anything the body can recognise and respond to. Not surprisingly, most drug prescriptions are written for two or more medications — the second drug usually being prescribed to counteract the side-effects of the first one, and if there is a third drug, this will almost certainly be written up in order to ameliorate the effects of the others. In a world where facing this type of challenge is a regular occurrence, it is little wonder that we have forgotten the elegant simplicity and effectiveness of natural ways. Little wonder, too, that it can take a while for us to reconnect with our own nature and reawaken our inner knowledge about what is best for ourselves.

Nature Cure charts this journey back towards full health and well-being, beginning in Chapter 2 with a full inventory of your health history in its widest possible sense. We then undertake a thorough assessment of your current state of health, happiness and physical well-being. Once you have opened your own health file, and become your own health detective, you are on the way to redressing any previous insults to the fullest possible health that is your birthright, and can move on through the book discovering more ways to enhance and augment your own well-being using all that Nature has to offer.

Introduction

When we look to the integrity of our experience, we see how bringing together body and mind in a unity of purpose provides us with a powerhouse of ideas and means to achieve our goals. This is why the use of imaging and visualisation techniques is as important a part of full health as dietary supplements or taking regular exercise. When we know ourselves, and can find peace, we have a wonderfully welcoming and stable centre around which to gather all the aspects of our life. When the body is working well and we experience happiness, then our everyday life becomes easier and more pleasurable. Symptoms of low energy and general malaise tend to disappear as we start to embody our life in all its aspects. Practical, health-enhancing measures become easier when we know the sense of them and do not divorce our thinking, conscious mind from the workings and needs of the body.

Being out in the natural world can sometimes be enough in itself to redress any minor health imbalance. The habit of taking a break by the sea, or a holiday in the sun, will often meet our inner need to bring those elements into our daily life. Taking a walk in the park, through a wood, or even along a leafy avenue seems to appeal to the delicate sense of balance within us, and can be a cure for headaches and other minor ills, as well as righting any feelings of being out-of-sorts. However sophisticated we become, there is no doubting our physical response to the sight of natural beauty whether it is a spectacular waterfall, a string of mountain peaks, or the first flowers of spring. We become touched in a place that is left uninspired by city vistas of uniform, squared buildings and shades of grey and stone. Our need to rest our eyes upon a gentle, alive, undulating landscape, and to feel our skin touched by the winds and warmed by the sun remains very much alive. It is as though being in nature allows some basic level of ourselves to resonate, vibrating in harmony as we recognise the majesty of our own beginnings, and all that we share in. This is as vital an aspect of full health as any other of our senses, awarenesses and abilities.

The Nature Cure philosophy takes an interesting view of healthcare. It maintains that we are constantly striving towards fuller health, and that our efforts can best be concentrated on facilitating, supporting and encouraging that move, rather than blocking it, ignoring it, misinterpreting and then suppressing the signs that the body gives us. Nature Cure embraces all aspects of our life because it recognises that sometimes what we need to balance ourselves is a specific remedy, and other times it may be restoring our own natural cycle and rhythms, or getting back in touch with 'the great outdoors' and reconnecting with our roots. Whether it is a need for social contact or a requirement for more roughage in the diet, a craving for vitamin C, or a lack of fresh air, Nature Cure recognises that only we ourselves know the answers to our own health needs, and can define the route back to full health.

All things exist in balance. The very fact of life on this planet is maintained due to a careful balance between the elements of earth, air, fire, water and spirit. If there was excess fire — if the sun burned too strongly — then life would not exist as we know it. Similarly, if there were 20 per cent more water here, the world would be completely changed, and our physical form would most likely be very different. Maintaining full health for our bodies means keeping a balance between the different elements. This same balance is needed in the rest of our lives to ensure not just the continuance of our physical well-being, but also the furtherance of our ideals, dreams and aspirations. We are not experiencing full health if we have ideal blood-pressure readings but are lonely and unhappy. Similarly, we can be slim and beautiful, but if we are frustrated and unable to express ourselves creatively, then we are not experiencing optimum health and well-being.

Our bodies are tremendously adaptable, and are always endeavouring to move towards ongoing health, but there is a limit. Junk food, chemical diets, atmospheric pollutants and emotional and physical stress all take their toll on the body's resources. The way of health is as much to do with prevention as it is with cure. If we are able to recognise our own needs, then we can make sure that we are able to respond to them. If there is a history of weakness in a particular area of your body or your life, then the gift of this discovery is that you know exactly where you need to channel your energy and focus your resources in order to strengthen and improve your health.

Making your ongoing health a priority in your life means making sure not to expose yourself to any unnecessary risks, learning how to preserve and maintain your strengths, and ensuring that no undue pressures are placed upon you. Staying well means staying happy, and doing everything within your power to ensure that you remain that way. Your nature will hold that vision of perfect health for you as a template, and the Natural world will support you in making your vision a reality.

Nature Cure

You are an amazing, self-regulating, self-healing organism, and want only the right environment and the right support to thrive and to experience absolute success. This means that given the chance, you can be healthy, happy, have all the energy you need and feel good.

Nature Cure is about a really useful system of healthcare that is mostly free and readily available to all of us. It is easy to use and has a myriad of applications, from keeping us well and happy to addressing specific health concerns. It is something we can all use every day of our lives to support our own constitutional strengths and face our individual health challenges. It is also a truly wonderful way to live because it honours the natural process within ourselves, and the role of Nature and the natural world. It is a practical way of harmony that respects our own personal balance, recognising that to interfere with that is not the route to well-being. Nature Cure methods always support, enhance and encourage the body's own inherent wisdom.

Understanding the philosophy of Nature Cure shows us how best we can use these myriad methods as prevention — to strengthen our own health — and as remedies. Essential to all healing is an appreciation of how the body works, and the many ways in which this can help us achieve optimum health and well-being. This means reaching beyond learning about your own anatomy, and discovering your own individual strengths and health challenges. It is also about fully living your life and that means enjoying it, taking responsibility for it, and sharing that with others. It doesn't mean that you can treat your health with less care than you would your motor car — responding only to its most basic needs, handing it over to the garage mechanic occasionally for a service, or when something seems to be going wrong.

Your health, well-being and happiness are intimately linked, and they are central to your life. You cannot be totally healthy when you are burdened with worry, nor completely happy when you are experiencing physical pain. Realising that we are the total of our experience is central to Nature Cure. It means that we might look to the personal world of our emotions for the root of any disharmony or unhappiness, or for a greater sense of balance in all our undertakings; or to the physical level to unearth dietary needs or allergies. It recognises that all our needs are equally important, and that the answers to our health concerns are always personal and individual.

Nature Cure maintains that your body is always working towards your own best health, and has an impressive and vital way of interpreting the signs and symptoms of ill-health. This allows us to distinguish between a Disease Crisis and a Healing Crisis. The former occurs when the body is unable to continue functioning at its best. It is a cry for assistance from our conscious awareness. This is what happens when the pain gets too bad, or we have to take to our beds for a few days, or when we cannot actually get up. To ignore this cry for help is a terrible thing. Simply switching it off by using pain-killers is no answer, merely a way to get some short-term relief. What the body needs at this time is for us to take a look at what has gone wrong, and what we may do to restore balance to our lives.

The body has a wonderful way to ensure that it maintains a balance between what we take in and what we put out. Appetite is at the front line of this mechanism, and our taste buds are the lucky arbiters of choice in this aspect of our lives. The presence in the diet of flavour enhancers, artificial and synthetic flavour substitutes and chemical taste-bud stimulants makes for a regular insult to these delicately-balanced bits. It is little wonder, then, that our taste buds can seem on occasion to let us down, and steer our desire away from natural foods.

Once in the system, the job of digestion is to sort, process, assimilate and then eliminate. If any one of these processes falls behind, it is easy to see how a degree of internal confusion can occur. Imagine that you feed yourself substances that the body is not able to recognise and does not know how to sort or process. This is what you do every time you take a genetically-altered, synthetically-copied or chemically-grown substance in your meals. When the body is stuck with something that it doesn't know how to process, it will endeavour to find a way, and failing that, will try to eliminate it from the system. It seems like such a waste of energy to spend all those resources on something that we know will not benefit us.

The body's routes of elimination need regular support and encouragement in order to keep them free and functioning well. Simple skills such as skin brushing (see page 148), taking regular air-baths (see page 148), and avoiding chemical anti-perspirants will improve the skin's ability to eliminate through its pores.

Dietary care and careful exercise will keep the bowel working well, and drinking enough water will support the work of the kidneys. The mucus membranes also respond well to dietary care, and the lungs can be helped by keeping a careful watch on environmental factors and making sure we use as much of their facility as we can. If you know that you have a weakness in a particular area of elimination, it makes sense to strengthen it as much as you are able and also to reinforce the body's other routes of elimination to let them share the burden.

Whenever we experience a crisis of disease, our first response needs to be to allow the body to heal itself as well as it can. Usually this means resting, so that vital energy is not used up in locomotion and movement but can be redirected to where it will be of most use. Resting physically frees up a lot of energy. Resting the digestive system does likewise, so switching to a very light, simple diet, or to a liquid or other fast makes sense. Reviewing how well your body is working — what eliminative routes need extra support, and what excessive loads may have pushed your body this far — will enable you to decide what best to do next. If this is a response to dietary excess, then a fast may well be the best choice, whereas a reaction to alcohol poisoning should point you in the direction of specific remedies, and the effects of a viral load may lead you to a more constitutional approach.

Whenever you let the body take the lead, it will do its best to return to full health as quickly as possible. This can involve a Healing Crisis — the point where the body is making its final push towards optimum health, and can create symptoms of unease while it loads the eliminative routes to their maximum. This is always followed by increased energy and renewed well-being.

The body will tend to heal itself from the inside out, and from the head down, following the course of health concerns back through time. This means that your most recent symptoms of ill health will be the first that are tackled, and that reaching back to deal with earlier insults will take a little more time. If you are resting and taking a natural course of action you can expect to see your current symptoms eased quite quickly, and will then need to choose whether you give your body the freedom to continue its healing work or switch back to normal, everyday life. Whichever you choose, the lessons learned can allow you to build for a healthier future.

By working with our own nature and the energies, elements and remedies that Nature makes available to us, we are able to work towards greater constitutional strength and heightened immune function. Whenever we respond wisely to the signs and symptoms that the body shows us, we take a step closer to full health.

We are a complete unit — a body that has a large head clearly placed on the top of it — and yet we do not connect our thoughts and feelings often enough with the way our body works. We take a huge step towards greater health when we recognise the totality of our experience, and integrate what we feel and see with what we perceive and know. In the words of the old song, your knee bone is most definitely connected to your thigh bone ... If your digestive system is working well, you will be getting the maximum nutrition from your meals and this will ensure among other things that any wounds heal quickly, your hair grows sufficiently long and luxuriant, your immune system will function well, and you will not experience tension headaches as the result of a sluggish bowel. If you are stressed and worrying, or if you feel as though your heart has been broken, your digestive system will not work well. How we feel affects the way the body works, and the way the body works affects how we feel.

Splitting off our head from our body is a relatively recent phenomenon. Hippocrates, the 'Father of modern medicine', spoke at length about the need to recognise the integrity of the individual, but these words seem to have been forgotten by the scientists of our day. Nature Cure practitioners honour the body's own self-regulating, self-adjusting and self-healing ability, recognising the importance of homeostasis. The concept of practising therapies which are directed towards releasing our inherent healing force, therefore aiding in the restoration of this homeostasis or equilibrium and reversing the disease process, is unique to Nature Cure. It is the only system of healthcare that carefully defines what is normal or natural for the body, and it limits its practices to reinforcing the person using only those methods.

Today many practitioners will disagree as to the extent or range of practices that can be considered natural or in harmony with the life purposes of each individual. Those methods and techniques described here form the core of Nature Cure in practice, and include some remedies and supplements that can be considered Nature's gifts to us. These include, for instance, flower remedies and essential oils. Any practices and therapies which violate the integrity of the individual in any way are not included here. Such practices include specialities such as acupuncture which routinely punctures or burns the skin, hypnosis, and homeopathy. These are separate systems of healthcare with their own laws and methods of cure.

Try Nature Cure for yourself, and see what a positive difference it will make to your life to be acting in so harmonious and direct a way to ensure your ongoing health, happiness and well-being.

Getting the Most from Nature Cure

This book is designed to introduce to you the concepts and practices of Nature Cure, and how best they can be built into a useful, practical form of healthcare for your own use. The individual chapters include advice on when to choose that form of cure, and how best to use it. Exercises and techniques are included to ensure that you can begin to use Nature Cure methods and remedies straight away.

Chapter 2 begins by reinforcing your position as your own Specialist Consultant and Chief Expert in your specialist subject: your life, health and well-being. The questions raised there will lead you towards being your own health detective, and getting a good fix on where you are right now in terms of your ongoing journey towards optimum health and happiness. It explores how you may best discover your own individual and unique recipe for well-being, and recognises the importance of factors such as contentment, spiritual awareness and values, as well as more practical concerns such as diet, exercise, counselling, etc.

Looking after ourselves, and living well, involves meeting a number of different needs, and sometimes simply recognising that these can have a profound effect upon our health. The way we handle stress, for example, and how we prioritise essentials such as time for relaxation and outdoor contact, can speak volumes about our ability to care for ourselves.

All the subsequent chapters will lead you to experience for yourself the wealth of natural resources and remedies that is available to you right now. Each chapter specialises in one area of natural healthcare, and they can all be dipped into or read from beginning to end. Every one should provide you with a myriad of different ideas to promote and enhance your own health and well-being. You can try them all — quite safely. You will soon find those with which you have a natural affinity.

Nature Cure will become a resource that is both exciting and comprehensive, as it guides you through the many ways in which natural remedies and harmony can work for you. All nature's methods can be used to form an effective line of defence against ill-health. Whether dealing with general matters like strengthening the immune system and the constitution, or addressing specific and immediate health concerns, Nature Cure's many practical applications will work gently and surely to encourage your body to right itself. This practical guide to staying well provides clear instructions for a full range of natural healthcare measures, as well as advice on making and using remedies.

All of these methods are embraced in an elegantly simple and practical philosophy of cure — Only Nature Heals. Often the best thing we can do for our own health is to stop interfering with it, and allow natural processes of vitality and renewal to take over. When we provide the right building blocks of food and nurture, experience the best physical and emotional atmosphere, and fulfil our needs for movement, elimination and self expression, we create good health.

Each chapter expands on these necessary elements and sets out a complete guide to working with your own health to achieve your goals for fulfilment, optimum energy levels, fitness and well-being.

Food is one of our strongest and most immediate medicines, and Chapter 3 focuses on our awareness of the medicinal and curative values of what we eat, as well as defining when other measures such as fasting and juice-diets can best be followed. General and specific exercise routines can remind us of the pleasures of movement and its importance in our lives — we can choose to focus on the sensuous or the energetic nature of dance and movement in order to meet a wealth of different physical needs. Whether you choose to support your health through activities and exercise, or through taking supplements or tissue salts to re-balance the system, the result is always one of enhancing your own self-regulating ability.

Our awareness of the actions of Spirit in our lives, and our duty of care towards our body-selves is as important to our everyday healthcare as the food we eat and the exercise we take. We can ensure that all we do takes place in an atmosphere of positive life enhancement — or we can decide not to bother. The choice is ours. Overall, if your focus is on what you may do to enhance and improve your general well-being, then you increase your ability to enjoy life.

This can mean eating the right foods to ensure optimum energy levels throughout the day, or using affirmations to assist in manifesting what you need. It can involve realising the need to feel sunlight touch your skin and scheduling time for this into your diary, or embarking upon a programme of self-help measures to revitalise your body. Whether you choose from the range of Hydrotherapy exercises, or elect for some of Nature's Gifts (essential oils, flower remedies, etc.,) each chapter sets out what you can expect to experience from each method. Each of the cures is explored in terms of why and how it works, when best to use it, the types of complaint it will work best with; and notes any safety measures to bear in mind.

Nature Cure places our experience within the context of nature, and is a hymn of praise to the myriad ways that the natural world can support and enhance our lives. It reminds us of the comprehensive range of solutions to all our everyday health concerns, and shows us how to bring some of the beauty of nature indoors. In harnessing the power of the elements, transforming simple ingredients into effective cures for all manner of ills, exploring our own inner healing, and adding medicinal plants to our diet we embrace the skills of managing our own healthcare in a safe, natural and effective way.

Our earliest written records speak of the abundance of ways that nature supports and enhances our health, and make much of the 'art of listening' — the importance of hearing the body's needs clearly in order that we may best respond to them. When Hippocrates spoke of the body's inherent ability to heal itself, he said it will always do so provided it is given the opportunity. Some 2,000 years later we still have access to the elements and the gifts of nature, and can work with natural methods to maintain optimum health. Our bodies have changed little in that time, and we can still use the simple cures that nature provides.

Living Naturally

Spending time out of doors provides us with the oxygen we need to think straight, and for our body to function well. It also touches some important part of ourselves that needs to feel the harmonious vibration that comes from sharing this space with other living things. It is very important to schedule time out of doors into our busy diaries in order to make sure that we attend to this vital aspect of our health and well-being.

Time spent dancing, moving and having fun, sharing our experiences with others and taking space for ourselves are all equally important aspects of our total well-being, yet these are less easy to define as therapies or practices, and therefore can often become marginalised in our life. Taking the time to determine exactly what we need in order to feel good in and about ourselves is the most useful thing we can do to forward our own nurturing and health. If dancing is your therapy, then make sure that you do it as often as you need to, and enjoy it thoroughly each time. If at this stage in your life you are crying out for some solitary space where you can just re-examine your priorities or simply be, then you *must* make this a priority and honour your own needs.

If you eat well, and allow food to be your medicine, and look to your needs in all other areas of your life, then you are giving yourself the greatest possible opportunity to be well and happy. And that is a good way to live.

If you look around you, you will usually find that all you might need is made available to you — and we can respond so profoundly to the gentlest touch. It doesn't need surgical intervention to heal a broken heart; it can sometimes respond to the simple, caring touch of another, or to a movement of spirit, or the sight of the first spring flowers. Often knowing the root of our discomfort will lead us to find its resolution, so time spent in plumbing our emotional depths and exploring our spiritual heritage and belief systems will all lead us toward being able to function more effectively, as well as being able to search out our own healing.

When we encounter imbalance within ourselves, we can treat ourselves with exquisite care and gentleness, encouraging our system to right itself, and giving whatever help is needed. There is always the opportunity within the natural world for us to experience optimum health and happiness. When additional help and support is needed, nature again provides it in the form of remedies that are taken from the natural world and concentrated so that we may use them more easily. It is good for us, though, to unlearn some of the bad habits of this century, and not reach for a tablet or a potion to cure our ills. Investing the time and energy to search out the level of our own disharmony, and how best to right that, is a gift of love to ourselves.

Following a natural lifestyle means that we are less likely to be thrown off balance in our daily lives. Each person is individual in the degree of care and expression that his or her different aspects require in order to remain healthy. Discovering what works best for you is your key to the future. If you know that you need eight hours sleep every night to function at your best, then make sure that you get it. If you cannot get through the week without some strenuous aerobic activity to bust your stress levels, then do not let yourself be seduced into disregarding this.

In the most general of terms, you need to discover whether you are at your best when rising late or early in the day. Whether you need to experience constancy in your personal habits, or if for you variety is the spice of life. Some people need to have a simple breakfast consisting of a piece of fruit or just a glass of juice, whereas others do best if they have a hot savoury meal at this time, to fire them up for the morning ahead. To remain ignorant of your own basic needs in these respects is to be negligent in your duty of care for yourself. Besides, discovering your own blueprint for optimum health and vitality is a richly rewarding and exciting journey.

Learn your own cycles of health, and you will discover the route to your own cures. Your most important and primary relationship is with yourself, yet we so rarely make time to be alone with ourselves and our innermost needs, thoughts, desires and dreams. Make a few minutes for yourself at the beginning and end of every day, and use this time to feel centred in your dreams for the future, and your present reality. Review the events of the day and how you are feeling.

Consider devotion and other spiritual values and how important they can be to you, and you will see a way to manifest them in your daily life.

Practically, it is important to allow yourself time for rest and renewal, so schedule breaks in your day for you to make the transition from one activity to another — e.g. at the end of the working day when switching into social gear, and before retiring at night.

Taking a shower can be a perfect opportunity to give yourself a loving all-over massage with the soapsuds; every drink can enhance your health, and you have tremendous power of choice over what you take into your world — through determining what you will read, watch and listen to, as well as selecting specific foods and nutrients.

Every day of your life is a precious gift that you have a purpose for, and you deserve to be able to fulfil that desire, and enjoy it to the utmost. Achieving this will be assisted by keeping your body well and happy, so eat five portions of fresh fruit and vegetables every day; exercise as much as you need to; allow yourself the support and encouragement you need from all areas of your world, and remember your place within the natural world and the changing of the seasons.

Chapter 2

INDIVIDUAL HEALTH

The journey to full health is one of the most exciting and rewarding adventures in life, and is tremendously empowering in terms of personal knowledge as well as increased energy and well-being. It is an area of your life on which you are a expert, with real insider knowledge. It is one of your own specialist subjects. It makes absolute sense to put your knowledge and expertise into practice, and this chapter is all about getting a clearer grasp on this most valuable asset, and reclaiming some of the secrets that your memory may be storing for you.

Health is a very personal thing. All humans share the same blueprint, but there are as many subtle and important differences, as there are people. Some have blue eyes, and some brown, some have dark hair with a tendency to grey, and others blonde hair with curls. The basics are the same, but the important details are different. Although we all have a digestive system that functions in a similar way, some of us can eat much more freely than others. We may have a tendency to put on weight or to be slim. The things that stimulate and benefit one person can overtax another, and some of us are better without *any* additional stimulation.

Determining your own basic constitutional picture enables you to work with your own best efforts to achieve optimum health for yourself. Your own recipe for full health will be unique to you. Although you may well share large elements of it with others, nobody else will have exactly the same needs or responses as you, and nobody else will attach the same meaning to it, because it will not be appropriate to them.

Nature Cure philosophy maintains that your body is doing its best for you right now. It is constantly moving towards full and total health. Your job is to learn how best to interpret its actions and meet its needs. Often this can mean simply getting out of the way and letting your body do what it knows how to do best — like generating its own hunger and food desires and managing its own elimination. Learning to dialogue with your body, and developing an appreciation of its basic needs, requires very little in terms of time or commitment, and can lead to a lifetime of improved health and well-being. The importance of this connection between your mind and your body cannot be overstated. It is one of your most effective tools in moving towards optimum health and happiness, and is the major way that you can create your own future.

Colds are an interesting example of Nature Cure at work. They obviously come at a time when the body needs to eliminate something, and is using the mucus membranes to do that. Supporting the body's own best efforts by easing the rest of its load makes the job easier. This means giving yourself plenty of rest and following a very light diet, so that the body does not need to work hard at all the labour of processing, digesting and assimilating foods, and can use its energy to speed up elimination. Increasing the effectiveness of other routes of elimination, like sweating, and drinking lots of water to help your kidneys rid the body of excess fluid, will also relieve the pressure on the mucus membranes.

Opening your own health file, as a place for all your knowledge about yourself and your health history, will enable you to clarify your own picture of well-being. It will make clearer your choices for the future, bring relevant memories to the surface, and shed light on any areas that are in need of a little extra help. This can be as clinical or as comprehensive as you choose to make it, and can become a major project while you clear your focus and prepare to take a new, streamlined look at your health and lifestyle.

Your own sense of well-being, your constitutional strengths, as well as areas where you need some additional support, are affected as much by what you think and feel, and your own likes and dislikes, as they are by more traditional factors such as your genetic make-up and heritage. This means that you have an amazing ability to transform your life with each new thought, each moment you experience, each movement you make, and with every breath you take.

Your Inheritance

You can chart your own recipe for full health and happiness through the health history of your family. Invariably there are family traits that come down through the generations, and it is not just physical factors that are influenced by heredity. Debate continues as to how much of our behaviour, thinking patterns, posture and other habits is influenced by what we learn as children, and how much is 'hard-wired'. Up till the age of five, we are permanently steeped in a rich growing medium that is full of family lore — we infuse a broad spectrum of information on everything from how to communicate to the best way to carry ourselves. Our learning faculties are so acute that we soak up all sorts of knowledge, and we function on a level that is not just verbal, so we also absorb a lot about emotions and feelings. This is when our body-typing skills are at their peak and we can sense and interpret what is going on from the most subtle interpretations of body language.

When a way of being, or perceiving, or an attitude or posture is learned very early in life, its influence on us is as great as if it had been genetically programmed. The distinct difference is that these learned factors are easier to relearn or resolve.

YOUR FAMILY TREE

Drawing your own family tree is a useful way of bringing together the many strands of genetic and other heritage that is relevant to your current health and well being. You will be able to bring to your conscious awareness a range of facts and information about your physical and emotional lineage, and this will show the type of template you are now living and working with. It is useful to paint as wide a picture as possible for each of the members of your family tree, and to include as many people and generations as you can. This can become a wonderful project that can be as wide ranging as you like, and may lead you to discover all sorts of interesting facts about your heritage. It is also a lovely gift to make to the generations that follow you.

Begin by collecting all the information that is available on those family members that you know about. You may find it easiest to draw out the basic family connections, and the conventional way to do this is on a large sheet of paper with lines running up and down through the generations, and from side to side to show partnerships and siblings. This will give you a skeleton which you can expand upon, embellish and decorate in whatever way you choose. Then you can begin to collate the additional information you want.

Consider health in the widest possible terms, and paint as broad a description as you can about each person. The facts that you need include the date and cause of death of your forbears, and the dates of birth and states of health of those who are still living. Older family members and friends will often be a good source of stories and anecdotes, and this can extend the scope of the project. Go beyond the more obvious facts. Did they like cats? Were they outdoors-types? Did they have strong feelings? What were their individual passions? Consider their character traits and scruples, whether they were hard-working, clever, demonstrative, etc. On the physical side, include data on how fertile they were, and smaller health factors such as whether they had good eyesight and hearing, etc., had a strong constitution or were prone to minor ailments. Find out whether they were happy, jovial types or prone to depression; whether they were outgoing or solitary. Include a photo or some form of sketch of how they looked.

It is valuable to think of the type of family you come from in terms of your potential for health and happiness. It is also useful to plot the way that family factors are inherited — you may look like one member of the family, for instance, and have a similar emotional make-up to another. We often exhibit the physical type of one parent, or side of the family, and the emotions of the other. Sometimes characteristics seem to skip one generation, or seem to disappear, only to re-emerge two or three generations later.

This, and the following information on your personal health history, should enable you to build a good picture of where you are now and where you come from. This is good information to have when becoming your own health detective, and will serve you in many ways.

Personal Health History

This is a full and often revealing story of your life to date. It may be necessary to ask others for some of the information you need to complete this, and it will almost certainly be thought-provoking as you bring to light health episodes from your past. It covers your emotional and psychological or energetic health, as well as that of your body, and will build into a comprehensive picture of your past.

The following form is a guide to the type of questions you need to ask yourself, and the general areas to explore. You may want to construct your own form, or use this one as a basis for your own case notes. Be as honest and comprehensive in your answers as possible, and add any additional details, or sections, that are relevant to your own health history.

Your Health Questionnaire

Note the date and time that you complete this, the season, and how you are feeling right now.

Have you ever:

- Had surgery — when and what for?
- Stayed in hospital — when and what for?
- Had any medical tests (X-rays, vaccines, given/received blood)?
- Broken any bones?
- Taken any:
  - prescription drugs?
  - long courses of medication?
  - over-the-counter medication e.g. laxatives?
  - other drugs?
  - supplements?
  - other remedies?
- Smoked cigarettes?

Have you had any of the following symptoms?

- Headaches
- Migraine
- Sinus troubles
- Dental caries
- Bleeding gums
- Hearing difficulties/earache or infections
- Neck/shoulder pain

Recurrent colds, sore throat
Chest pain/ difficulty breathing
Emotional disturbances
Depression
Skin trouble
Swellings
Back pain
Foot problems — fallen arches, ingrown toenails, etc.
Menstrual difficulties
Digestive concerns — indigestion etc.
Bowel complaints — constipation, diarrhoea, etc.
Other physical concerns

Were you breast-fed?
Did you have brothers and sisters — what is their health like?
What was home like?
Did you have vaccinations?
Were you a strong, healthy child?
Did you experience all the common childhood diseases, e.g. mumps, measles, etc.?
Did you play a lot?
Are your memories happy ones?
Do you remember being warm or cold whilst growing up?
Are your memories spread throughout the year, or do they tend to be seasonally-based?

How was adolescence?
Did you: get acne/become very emotional/turn inwards/become extrovert/rebel against authority etc.?
Did you develop friendships and relationships easily?
Did you enjoy school?

When was your first period?
What sanitary products did you use?
When and how did you become sexually active?
How many partners have you had?
Do you enjoy sex?
When was your first orgasm?
What form of contraception did you use?
Any pregnancies?

Any: on-going health concerns or trends?
difficulties that have remained with you?
events or incidents that have coloured your experience or changed you?

What is your strongest body-related memory?

What is your earliest memory?

What is your philosophy of health?

You may find that you feel a need to focus on a particular time in your past, or a specific event in order to review the past thoroughly and make a complete picture. There is no limit to the amount of information you can gather to make this health file as comprehensive as it needs to be. Often, compiling the facts and remembering the events will bring feelings and emotions to the fore, and the work can be very healing in itself. Spending this much time honouring your past is also a wonderful gift to be making to yourself, and the process can be transformational.

In our society we tend not to pay too much attention to this inner work, and there is often little time for reflection on our health history. Visits to allopathic practitioners seldom allow time for individuals to piece together their own health jigsaw, let alone for the reverie that allows insights and intuition to frame the picture, or fill in any gaps. Take all the time that you need now in order to complete this vital piece of your health file.

YOUR HEALTH TODAY

Your health and happiness is about more than how you are feeling physically. Your lifestyle, habits, occupation, emotional contentment and a range of other factors affect the quality of your experience. Consider the following factors to see how rounded is your current choice of lifestyle, and to help you identify any areas of potential change. It may be that you could alter the focus of your leisure time, or place more emphasis on your own nurturing. Use the following questions as a guide, and include any areas of special interest or relevance to yourself and your own life.

Note the date and time that you complete this, the season, and how you are feeling right now.

Are you happy?
Do you find this exploration exciting?
Do you feel comfortable right now?

Do you:
- enjoy your life?
- think diet is important to your health?
- sleep regularly? easily? well? deeply?
- dream often? ever have nightmares?
- awake refreshed?

Do you:
have good overall energy levels?
have any hobbies?

How much time do you:
spend with your hobbies each week?
spend each day watching television?
spend outdoors each week?

How do you have fun, and how much time do you spend doing this each week?

Do you have a personal computer?
How long do you spend on it each day?

Do you have a faith, a religion, or spiritual beliefs?

Do you work?

Are you in a relationship?
Do you have a good social life?
Are you close to your family?
Do you feel supported by family and friends?
Are you happy spending time alone?

Do you use anti-perspirants?
Do you use anti-dandruff shampoo?

How much exercise do you take each week?
What sort?
For how long?
How do you feel afterwards?
How often do you go for a walk?
Do you enjoy spending time in nature?

Do you:

feel comfortable in yourself?
like your body?
have a favourite time of year?
feel well?
think you have enough energy when you need it?
express yourself creatively?
honour what is sacred in your life?
spend time in meditation or contemplation?
have enough time for yourself?
express your anger easily?
feel sympathy for yourself and others when appropriate?
have the ability to walk away from negative situations or habit patterns?
often feel enthusiastic and positive about your life?
consider yourself to be good at looking after yourself?
deal easily with your emotions and those of others?
have enough structure in your life?
feel prosperous and enriched?
fulfil your own promise?

What is the aspect of your body that needs most care and support?
What is your strongest physical asset?

Interpreting the answers to your questions will become easier when you review the questionnaire as a whole. There are no right or wrong answers, and no points to be scored in any place. You are looking for your own sense of balance, and what is natural and healthy for you. This questionnaire will help reveal to you any areas of your life that currently appear to be either impoverished or under-energised. If your review shows that you spend too much time working, or sitting at a computer screen or watching television, and seldom take a walk in the sunshine, or play, or have a good laugh, then the remedy is obvious. Shifting your priorities can become easier once you have a clear picture of what needs to change.

You may also like to consider factors such as how much you embrace the natural world, and/or are surrounded by artificial, synthetic factors, and whether you feel this fosters good health. This part of your file should be thought provoking, and may lead you to make some decisions about enriching your experience in some way, perhaps undertaking a course of study, or including more creative forms or means of expression. Whatever actions you take, make sure that you do something to redress any imbalance that you can see when you look at this review of your life.

This may be the first time you will have spent considering these issues, and may also be your first opportunity to clearly identify what works in your life, and what doesn't. The final questions are very useful in pinpointing the steps you need to take immediately: how you can best build on your strongest asset, and what measures you need to take to ensure that the part of you that needs most help gets it. This may mean acknowledging that you have a weak digestion, and making sure that you feed yourself carefully, choosing warm foods and eating in a relaxing environment; or recognising a sluggish system, and remedying that with regular exercise and hydrotherapy techniques.

All this new information should fit together with the information you gathered in your health history to give you quite a detailed picture of your current health. The more you are able to define your health needs, the easier it is to meet them in appropriate, natural, supportive ways. Often this does not even call for a remedy or a cure, but a yet simpler shift in focus, or time commitment, or habit pattern. Understanding more about the nature of your own situation enables you to piece together your own unique recipe for full health and happiness.

Your Body's Language

One of the ways that your body has of communicating is through the signs and symptoms of ill-health. It is said that the body speaks with the voice of the soul, and it is not hard to see that this could be so, in the simple, direct way that the body has of doing things.

There are many different ways to look at the body's ailments, including considering whether they are drawing our attention to a physical site that is in need of care, or to an area of our lives that is in need of attention. If, for instance, you often experience colds and flu symptoms, think about why that is. Could it be that there is a need for you to take some rest, and that a few days alone and taking a break would benefit you? If your cold is making your head all stuffed up, perhaps there is a need to cry to relieve the pressure, or to get some fresh air or new ideas into your life, or to take some measures to reinforce your immune system and strengthen yourself generally. It doesn't make any sense to try to divorce the way we feel physically from what is going on in the rest of our lives, and so the obvious way to treat stubborn or recurring health concerns is to widen our approach to include other aspects of our experience. If you are stuck in a cycle of the same symptoms reappearing, and responding to them using the same type of remedy, then perhaps it is time to try a broader approach.

If your cold always leaves you with congested sinuses, or with a sore throat, or breathing difficulties, why is that? Is this area of your body weakened in some way? Your question must be how best can you strengthen and heal it — and the answer has to be in your *life*, not just in your head and neck. Taking the right natural remedy will effect a straightforward cure, and the effectiveness of this can be enhanced by tackling any dysfunction in this area of your life. The throat area corresponds to the energy of communication, and it is influenced by and affected by the quality and quantity of your communications, how well they are received, and the way that you feel about this.

Consult the following chart for some ideas about how physical location can be linked to motivations and areas of life. It is a tremendously healing experience to broaden your focus in such a way, and to harness all your skills and energies for the purpose of rebalancing your life. It may seem strange at first to consider how you feel emotionally, or what you are doing with your time in response to a recurrent physical concern, but it will result in a comprehensive cure that re-energises you on many levels, as well as healing your body.

Area of Body	Area of Life/Motivation
Head	Inspiration — that which inspires us intellectually and spiritually; our link with the greater self, and the way we perceive that.
Throat	Communication — the quality and quantity of our contact within ourselves, and our own inner dialogue; how well we bridge the gap between head and heart. Communication with others.
Chest	The emotions and our ability to love — ourselves, one another, and all aspects of creation. Our capacity for being the greatest that we can be.
Trunk	Courage and physical strength — how we find our way in the world, and our sense of personal integrity. The centre of our physical form, and a place of balance for every level of our being.
Pelvis	Creativity and sexuality — the way we honour and express these energies. Containment, and how we may come to experience that. Our sense of stability and the seat of physical energy.
Spine	Our main means of support — whether that manifests itself in our life through letting others in and seeking out what we need. Remaining constant whilst enabling a flow of energy to enter and leave every aspect of life.
Limbs	The ability to move and to do. Where we are going in life, and what we are doing on our journey. Our absolute ability to move from one place to another, and to achieve the extraordinary.

These general energies will manifest themselves in different ways, and will affect each person differently. Building your own vocabulary of physical signs and symptoms will enable you to tailor your responses appropriately.

Different body areas respond well to different remedies and other natural techniques, and you can find further information on all of these in the following chapters. The herb red sage, for instance, is a wonderful cure for sore throats and stiff necks, having a special affinity with this area of the body. Toning and other techniques which express feelings and move energy out of the body are wonderfully effective with stubborn digestive and joint complaints like arthritis. Dance and Chi exercises can be an effective choice for spinal concerns.

Of course, these can only be ideas to guide you in your search for a deeper dialogue within yourself. You may like to find some ways to communicate directly and specifically with your body, and find out what direction it is seeking to guide you in, and what it is trying to say. One lovely way to start deepening this relationship is to give something to this aspect of yourself. An obvious choice is to use the language of touch, when you can convey love, care and nurturing in a warm and safe way. Simply placing your hands on a part of your body that is not usually held in this way will convey feelings of warmth and support. You can use a warmed massage oil to gently stroke and get to know your body better, or do this including a few drops of an essential oil to reinforce a therapeutic or other desired effect. Taking yourself for a professional therapeutic massage or aromatherapy treatment might be another way to deepen this connection. See also page 109 for directions on self-massage.

Sometimes you can 'hear' the voice of your body-self if you simply listen. It can come when you empty your mind of other thoughts and the busyness of everyday life. Time spent in reflection, contemplation or meditation can allow your inner wisdom to bubble up inside you and inform your mind. This can also become a dialogue if you choose to focus your energy on a question or on an area of your life that is in need of some clarity or a wider vision. Making this a regular part of your life is a great act of generosity to yourself.

Considering Cause and Effect

It is important to look at the many levels of our experience, and to consider the different ways in which we can respond to things. Having realised that our health is not separate from the way we live our lives, we can look at the way actions and events will influence our physical responses. It is not uncommon for hard workers to experience migraine headaches at the weekends, when they begin to relax and the body is then able to do whatever it needs to — whether that is drawing attention to that area or simply evidencing the build-up of stress and tension that has occurred through the week. Similarly, those who stop smoking may develop a cough, as the body is at last able to rid itself of some of the accumulation in the lungs.

If your health concerns follow a pattern, it may be useful to look at external events, as well as your own inner timing, to see whether there are any clues there. Obvious inner cycles include the four-week menstrual cycle and the three, six and twelve week immune cycles. External factors can include factors as diverse as visits from your mother to illnesses elsewhere in your family or social circle. It is worth looking at all the circumstances surrounding any episode of ill health, particularly if it is a recurrent complaint, and piecing together the common elements. It is invariably a combination of things that can come together to push the body too far — perhaps dietary stress combined with an unpleasant or stressful task, or a shock or unfinished business when there is a sudden cold snap in the weather, *and* you haven't had enough sleep.

Sometimes the reappearance of an old, familiar health concern can simply be your body reminding you that you need to be in another place, or to take some time for yourself, away from the needs and concerns of others. We seldom prioritise time spent on our own, healing and caring for ourselves, but we all need it. Whatever the reasons we discover, it is important to trust the lead that the body gives, and to find ways to follow it.

The Need for Balance

A lot of physical energy is involved in the constant work of achieving balance. Your body needs to balance your energy requirements with your energy output, and hunger is one of the tools involved in maintaining this mechanism at an optimum level. Your temperature needs to remain within fairly tight limits — warm enough to keep you alive, but not too warm or damage occurs. Water levels are crucial to ensure that there is sufficient in the system to bathe it in a health-giving solution, and to carry water-soluble waste from the body. The range of functions that the body copes with quite independently of our conscious thought is awesome.

It is also good to practise balance in our conscious activities, so there is a symmetry between what we do consciously and what is occurring without our constant conscious appreciation. It makes sense to work out how best to balance our needs and desires, our activities and pursuits, and our social and solitary requirements.

Natural healing systems from all around our planet use different ways to assess the balance of our health. There are many different philosophies of healthcare, as there are in other areas of life. These can offer valuable insights into the way we look at our health, and where we may look to rebalance any disharmony. Consider the following brief points, and whether they are relevant to you.

The Chinese and other Asian systems consider whether a person and a complaint are hot or cold, empty or full, stagnant or fluid, stuck or over-flexible. Pan-global Shamanic teachings bring in the elements: does it feel fluid like water, strong like fire, fast and light like the air, or solid and constant like the earth? Does it move like the wind, have feline qualities, remind you of an animal or a bird? How does it feel emotionally — does it remind you of any past event, any person you know, any other time you have felt like this? Does it feel cool, like glass or metal, or warm and textured like velvet? The more ways you can understand your feelings and sensations, the more complete your experience, and the closer you are to well-being.

Whatever information you can gain can be developed and expanded upon — what colour is the velvet? where does the cat live? etc. All of this brings remarkable insights and the healing journeys begun can be quite extraordinary.

Working in this way opens up a range of different avenues for you to explore, and involves all of you: your imagination and your abilities to envision your life, your feelings and sensations, your senses and your heart, as well as your physical symptoms.

Whenever you are considering your health, it is important to also consider what is happening in the world outside of yourself: in your social circle and within your family; in your working relationships with colleagues, and those with other associates; and also outside of your window in the world of nature. Different seasons represent changing points in the cycle of the year, and can influence the way your body behaves and how you feel. Everyone notices how the sap seems to rise within as Spring bursts forth with its new growth and early flowers, and who can fail to feel a lightening in the heart when they see swallows flying across a clear blue sky?

We are a part of nature, and a part of our surroundings, and it is easy to see how we may become distressed, unbalanced or unwell by distancing ourselves from our home in this way.

Finding the root cause of any disharmony will enable you to rebalance yourself, and to take whatever actions are necessary in order to promote your own well-being. Another way to look at this is to find the level of any distress. You may feel it to be based in your body in a specific location or more generally, in your emotional world, your mind, your heart, your spirit, or you may feel yourself to be cut off from your energy, or your soul. Any of these are valid if you feel them. They also clearly point you towards the level on which you may need to work in order to resolve them and rebalance yourself.

Having brought many different aspects of yourself together in the search for your own optimum health, you have experienced how effective it can be to work with a unity of purpose, and to focus on your own healing. Now that you know and have used that ability, we can go on to look at the vast armoury of help and assistance that you can call upon to enhance and support your new-found sense of harmony.

Counselling

Self-counselling techniques are among the most creative problem-solving tools you will ever use. They are excellent because they confirm the belief that you yourself know what is the best course of action to take in any given situation, whether that is following a specific form of cure, or the direction or area in which to look for a remedy, and whether outside assistance is required.

We all tend to feel most at ease with a particular form of communication: written, visual or verbal. Work out for yourself what feels best, what you feel most at ease with, and use that to counsel yourself. If you feel you can understand things most clearly when they are written down, take some time to yourself, focus on your concerns, and write them down in the form of a letter. Read it through, and when you are sure that your letter is complete and contains all the aspects that are important and your desires for the best possible outcome, seal the letter in an envelope and post it to yourself. Once it is gone from your hands into the postal system, there is a wonderful sense of release, and when the letter arrives for you a day or two later, you will find yourself able to read it with a renewed sense of objectivity.

Another useful way to work with feelings is to keep a daily journal. Choose a special book or pad of paper to record the events of your life, and choose a time when you will do it every day. Keeping to a regular time is important, because you can develop a habit of keeping that time aside for yourself, when you are free to be your most creative and expressive, and know that you will have time for your emotional world and your innermost feelings. Record everything that you want to in your journal, in whatever way you choose, and then at the end of each week, make some time to sit and look back at the week you have just lived. See how good you feel about making time for yourself, and recording your life in this way, and note some of the changes and patterns that you have experienced. This may also give you an opportunity to discover new things about yourself, and to realise some abilities that you had not recognised previously. You may also see how you deal with worries and concerns, and what happens to them when you deal with them in different ways.

People who like to express themselves verbally may enjoy talking to themselves about their concerns, or speaking them into a tape that can then be played back and listened to dispassionately. A wonderful way of using this ability is to identify a range of different parts or aspects of yourself, and give each one of them a voice. Imagine all the characters that you can 'hear' speaking inside your head anyway — there might be a critic, who makes lots of judgements about things; an innocent, who likes to play and have fun; a worrier, warrior, rescuer, victim; you might hear the voice of a parent or someone you know, a Wise One — the list of possibilities is endless. Identify some of your own characters, and give them a voice. Make some ground rules for yourself — perhaps that only one 'voice' can speak at any one time, or that there is a Chairperson, and simply allow some truths to be spoken. It is amazing how effective this simple technique can be, in terms of identifying aspects of ourselves that need some form of expression, voicing feelings and thoughts that might otherwise have been left unsaid, and generally embracing the reality of our own inner world.

Voicing something in this way can relieve a lot of internal pressure, and the sense of relief can be quite remarkable. This sort of dialogue is something you can do whenever you feel the need to, or schedule into your diary for a weekly session.

People with a strong visual sense may like to draw or paint how they are feeling right now; or if this seems a little daunting, what about making some kind of visual image of your body, or your home, or your emotional world. Whatever you draw, paint, design or make, honour it in some way, and go back to it later with your analytical self — determine what aspects are there in strength, and those that are lighter, or absent. See what the work is really saying and define how it could be augmented in order to be more in balance and harmonious.

Whatever your best sense is, that is going to be your greatest helper, so it makes sense to make the most of it. If you feel things most strongly in your body, then work with your body to express, release and change them, and then bring in your mind to aid your understanding. Dance, movement and exercise are all good ways of working with this type of body-sense.

A quick problem-solving technique that was taught me by the Psychic Betty Balcombe is to draw a triangle on a piece of paper, with a one- or two-word description of the difficulty in the middle of the triangle. On the left, write down all the things that led to this situation — be as comprehensive as you can, and include all the points that you feel are relevant, however small they may be. When you have finished that list, write down all the possible outcomes on the right of the triangle. Be as imaginative and inventive as you wish, but be sure to include all the realistic options too, no matter how un-inspiring they may seem. Leave your work for a short time and take a break. When you return to it, see if there is anything else that you need to add. If not, review the whole thing, and you should find that your way forward, the best solution for you, becomes clear. Write this at the bottom of your triangle, and see how this feels. You do not need to act on it right away; you can just 'try it on for size' for a while.

List-making is a useful way to clarify what is in your mind and in your heart — or to get a clearer view of all the contributing factors. Making your lists in columns is a way to weigh the benefits of one side of the argument against the other, and you might also try writing your lists in a circle, or in free-form anywhere on a page, and then connecting up the bits that relate to each other. Let your imagination guide you.

It may seem trite to say that all problems are really challenges, and that the solutions are there for us. If we believe in our own basic goodness, and the presence of any greater self, guide, gods, love, or creative source, then we can release the fear that often comes associated with problems, and see them in a new light. Imagine if one of the things you needed to do while you are here is learn some lessons about specific areas of your life, then surmounting challenges and discovering your own problem-solving skills would be a good way to do that. We have available to us all that we need in order to grow, and one of our biggest challenges is in believing that.

A Healthy Future

Defining your own health goals will be much easier now that you have a clear and full picture of your current health needs. Your own individual strengths and challenges should be clearer to you, and you will also have begun to develop your inner communications, enabling you to find the source of any health concerns, and the right recipe to remedy them. The work you have done in discovering your capabilities, uncovering your past experiences and defining the way you feel right now will have cleared a path that should be easier to follow into your future.

All the information that you have gathered whilst working through this chapter will form the basis of how you approach your health needs and concerns from now on. You will have a vast armoury of different approaches to choose from that your body will have a natural affinity with, and that are all supportive and health-enhancing. Choosing a remedy or cure from another part of the natural world only reinforces your connections with your own nature, and is a safe and effective choice for all manner of health concerns.

Making good plans for the future means making today as good as it can be. This means balancing your needs with the best possible care, and knowing when to stretch yourself, and when to rest. It means being able to respond to your changing self in the most appropriate way, and drawing together all your many skills and attributes to ensure that one of your most basic and prized possessions — your health — is always a prime concern. This does not mean becoming obsessional about healthcare, but it does involve realising your duty of care to yourself, honouring your position as prime carer, and looking after yourself.

Once you have defined your own picture of full health, use every skill you have at your disposal to make it reality. Use visualisation techniques, affirmations, your creativity and your physical abilities too. Harness all your available energy to achieve full health. Plan the easiest, best and most enjoyable way to reach your goal, and structure it into achievable steps. Reward yourself appropriately when you achieve each one. Picture yourself living your life the best way you can, and behave as much as possible as though that were already so.

What you have read about here, and throughout this book, should enable you to fulfil your role of personal primary health-care provider in a natural, safe way that is effective and often pleasing. The remedies and cures mean that you will be able to treat yourself well whenever there is a symptom of unease or imbalance, and your knowledge of yourself and your own health requirements will enable you to choose wisely. Regaining control of your own happiness and healthcare is a remarkably healing action in itself, and will lead you forward to create your own future well-being.

Chapter 3

FOOD AND DRINK

We are, quite literally, what we eat. Each piece of food that we consume provides us with the materials we need to renew and repair ourselves, as well as supplying us with energy. Every part of the body is involved in a constant process of repair and renewal, and so we are fashioned from the very materials that we take in. A sobering thought, and one that reminds us that if we are giving the gift of life in our meals, then we benefit most if these are of the highest possible quality, carefully stored, prepared and offered with love.

The foods we choose provide us with the tools for ongoing good health: they are our natural medicine, and a powerful good health habit. Simple measures like ensuring you eat the best food you can, at regular intervals, and in good surroundings, mean that you are enhancing your health at every opportunity. Good food is like money in the bank of your constitutional well-being. These days there is much controversy as to what good food really is. The variety of foodstuffs we encounter as consumers is more daunting than ever, and more so now that genetically altered foods are readily available and cropping up in all sorts of strange places.

Food is the only way of providing your body with the physical energy it needs. Your body needs regular fuel in order to stay well, awake, and able to move around. Some simple measures can ensure that you are getting the most from your food:

- Plan to have three mealtimes every day, and make these as regular as possible. This way your body knows when it will be getting its next energy boost, and can plan accordingly.
- Let hunger guide you, and never force yourself to eat if you do not have an appetite. Leave enough time between meals for proper digestion — 2 hours between snacks, 4 hours between larger meals.
- Use meals as a special time when you can focus on your own positive nourishment.
- Be sociable when you eat if you can find good company; otherwise, enjoy your own company and savour the benefits of being good to yourself.
- Always eat sitting down, so that your body doesn't have to expend energy to do much else beyond enjoying its own nourishment.
- Eat foods that you like. Experiment with different tastes and flavours to broaden your palate and please your taste buds.
- Eat a variety of different foods. This is one of the best ways to avoid becoming bored, and makes sure that you will get a wide range of nutrients.
- Pay attention to your emotions. Do not eat when you are feeling angry or upset; attend to your feelings instead.
- Learn the effects of different foods in your body. Hot foods will raise your temperature, but there is much more to food than its thermal effects. Foods have different energising

qualities and medicinal effects as well as tastes, and their colour and appearance will also have an effect on you. Chillies will tend to stir you up, and carbohydrates will relax you, but every body reacts differently.

- Do all that you can to enhance your digestion. Make sure you chew food sufficiently, especially carbohydrates, and remain relaxed and calm during your meal and for a short time afterwards. Do not put out your digestive fire by eating or drinking anything too cold, and do not underestimate the effect of your surroundings. Watching a bad news programme will not benefit or enable your digestion; neither will anything too violent or loud.

> Gently stimulate your appetite by peeling a ½-inch piece of fresh ginger root and adding to a cup of boiling water. Sip slowly while still warm, and take 20–30 minutes before mealtime. Keeping regular mealtimes will also encourage your body. Adding a little fresh or dried ginger to the meal itself will heighten digestion and please your taste buds.

All food can be divided into certain basic groups:

Protein: this comes from animals and their products (cheese, eggs, milk); and from foods that provide protein when mixed together, e.g. nuts and seeds, beans and pulses, and grains.

Your body needs protein to repair itself and to make new growth. It is a good idea to eat some protein every day, and only small amounts are necessary for full health. Experiment with the full range of protein sources to ensure a wide variety in the diet, and to offer plenty of alternatives to animal protein.

Carbohydrates: these are starches like bread, potatoes, rice and pasta; sugars like those in fruit and milk, and fibre from vegetables, pulses, seeds and beans.

Carbohydrates provide your body with the energy it needs. These foods need to form the bulk of the diet. Aim to form each meal around the carbohydrate content, giving it centre stage, and choose as wide a range as possible in order to reduce any dependence on wheat.

Fats: these include dairy products, nuts and seeds and their oils, and vegetable oils as well as fish and fish oils. Fat is also found in beans and pulses.

Fats are necessary for the absorption of some nutrients, and provide some energy, insulation and protection. They are needed in quite small doses, and keep the body 'oiled'. Without doubt the best source of fat in the diet is that of vegetable origin, and Olive Oil is the tastiest and most health-enhancing. Do not be tempted to switch from butter to margarine; small amounts of butter are better for you than the range of chemicals and processed products in margarines, the list of which will usually not even fit across the lid of the tub, but have to be printed around its perimeter!

Vitamins, Minerals and **Trace Elements** are also to be found in foods. These are micro-elements that are essential to life and the proper functioning of the whole body. (See Nutritional Supplements, page 186.) Foods that are rich in these individual elements need to form a large part of your diet. The word 'vitamin' describes something that is essential to life, and these and other micro-nutrients such as minerals are present in theory in all the fresh fruit and vegetables that we eat. You need some of these every day to stay well.

This table shows some of the major actions and sources of a range of vitamins and minerals.

Vitamin/Mineral	Actions	Sources
Vitamin A	Important anti-oxidant. Essential for normal vision, healthy skin and other tissue	Sweet potato, carrot, squash and pumpkin, mango and all yellow-pigmented fruits and vegetables
Vitamin B complex	A range of actions including nervous system function, protein utilisation, liver health, carbohydrate digestion, fertility	Yeast, whole grains, green vegetables, eggs, nuts and animal products
Vitamin C	Vital anti-oxidant. Important to all wound healing, and the health of every body cell. Key to a healthy immune system	Fresh raw fruit and vegetables especially citrus fruits, parsley, black-currants, broccoli

Vitamin/Mineral	Actions	Sources
Vitamin D	Necessary for the formation of healthy teeth and bones and for calcium use	Sunlight. Dietary sources include sunflower seeds, eggs, butter, milk and fish liver oils
Vitamin E	Anti-ageing vitamin. Key to muscle function, fertility and skin health	Green vegetables, vegetable oils, nuts, wheat germ
Vitamin K	Vital to clotting of the blood, involved in the prevention of osteoporosis	Green leafy vegetables. This is synthesised in the gastro-intestinal tract
Minerals:		
Calcium	Essential to healthy teeth and bones, and to prevent osteoporosis and speed wound healing	Sesame seeds, tofu, kelp, nettles, dairy products and tinned fish
Magnesium	Involved in all muscle activity	Millet, soybeans, nuts, fresh vegetables
Potassium	Intimately involved with magnesium and vital to maintaining the body's acid balances	Most herbs, kelp, sunflower seeds, wheatgerm, bananas
Iodine	Necessary for proper metabolism and maintenance of energy levels	Kelp, fish, yoghurt, seaweeds and sea vegetables, and all produce grown near the sea

Vitamin/Mineral	Actions	Sources
Iron	Carries oxygen around the body and is important to the immune system. Women need to replenish their monthly loss	Blackstrap molasses, wheatgerm, parsley, apricots, raspberries, soya
Manganese	Vital to metabolism; aids the nervous system and full digestion	Wheatgerm, brown rice, all dark green leafy vegetables, egg yolks, pineapple, beetroot and blueberries
Zinc	Multiple synergistic actions within the body, regulates appetite, skin healing and the nervous system	Brewer's yeast, pumpkin and sunflower seeds, green vegetables and oysters

Foods also have medicinal and energetic qualities, e.g. garlic is a powerful antibiotic, and ginger will stimulate and warm your digestive system. Taking another look at everyday foods will lead you to discover a range of health-giving properties, for example:

Symptoms of gout can be relieved as much by what you do *not* eat as by what you do. Consider removing black pepper, alcohol, red meat and wheat from the diet, and eating fresh black cherries or taking their juice with as many meals as possible. These counter-effect the acid condition and bring speedy relief.

- Figs are a good laxative.
- Cranberries are an excellent urinary tract cleanser — useful in the treatment of cystitis.
- Cucumber removes uric acid from the blood, acts as a mild diuretic and is cooling in the summer.
- Lettuce reduces insomnia and encourages sound sleep.
- Beetroot is a liver tonic.
- Garlic stimulates your body's immune responses.
- Dates and raspberries both contain chemicals similar to aspirin.
- Bananas and other high potassium fruits may help prevent gastric ulcers.

Vitamin C has a wonderfully healing effect within the body, and will assist your immune system to resist opportunistic infection. Make sure you take extra amounts of this key vitamin during the cold and flu season. It is also useful if you bruise easily, if wounds or minor cuts take a long time to heal, and if your gums have a tendency to bleed. Consider taking a supplement if your needs seem to be great, or step up the amount of fresh fruit and raw vegetables that you eat. Vitamin C is available in powder form, and this makes an excellent skin-healing preparation when mixed with a little water and sprayed or painted on.

It is worthwhile being adventurous with your diet and adding some more uncommon foods to increase the variety of your mealtimes, and also to provide their health-giving elements.

Sea vegetables and **seaweeds** are very tasty, and excellent sources of minerals, especially iodine, so necessary for a good metabolism. These are used extensively in Oriental cuisine, and may be found, dried, in health food shops and Oriental food stores. They are available in packet form and usually have clear instructions on the labels. Look for Nori, sold in sheets or in flakes, and excellent for wrapping rice bundles, toasting and adding to vegetable and rice dishes, or just to sprinkle on to any savoury meal. Kombu is an excellent thickener, useful for adding to sauces and composite meals, and will also reduce the gas potential of all beans and pulses. Wakame is very tasty if soaked first, then cut into small pieces and added to salads. Carrageen can be ground and sprinkled over any dish, sweet or savoury, or used for its gelatinous quality in sweets and fruit jellies.

Mung beans are an excellent source of protein, and are very easy to digest. They have a wonderfully cleansing effect on the pelvis, and will clear any bowel congestion. They can be eaten as a soup or stew by simply boiling them up, or sprouted and added to salads, sandwiches, and a host of meals.

Constipation and pelvic congestion can be relieved within two days by focusing on Mung beans in the diet. Soak them overnight in cold water, then rinse well and add to twice their volume of water. Bring to the boil, and then simmer until the beans have all softened and broken. Add some crushed garlic and fresh ginger root to the pot and cook for a further five minutes, then eat with rice and a teaspoon of olive oil. Add some chopped coriander leaves or a teaspoon of the ground seeds to further enhance the effects.

Coriander or Cilantro leaves are an excellent addition to any meal. They have a cooling, soothing effect on digestion, and help a range of functions from bladder activity to eyesight clarity. A small spoonful taken every day is a good preventative measure.

Sesame Seeds are a rich source of calcium, so necessary to the health of the teeth and bones, and an important element for women as we grow towards the menopause and beyond. These can be ground into flour to add to all home baking, and appear in shops as Tahini, a savoury spread akin to peanut butter; Halva, a sweet made of sesame seeds, honey, and nuts or flavourings; and Gomasio, a mixture of the seeds and sea salt that can be used in place of salt at the table, and adds a new flavour to foods just before serving.

Soya is an excellent alternative source of protein and other nutrients, and is supremely versatile. Substitute Soya milk for cow's milk to enjoy a full range of meals whilst taking a break from over-reliance on dairy products. Include the beans in dishes to reduce the amount of animal protein you cook with. The bean curd, tofu, can be served in any number of ways, from creamed as a dip to marinated and added to stir-fry.

Grains are now available in an amazing range and variety, and these provide a change of flavour, a good carbohydrate source, and an alternative to any over-reliance on wheat. Consider millet, buckwheat, soya, rye, amaranth, barley and rice.

> If diarrhoea is a problem, consider eating a plain Matzo cracker and drinking small amounts of diluted and warmed apple juice. The combination of starch and sugar is an excellent binder for the whole digestive tract, and symptoms should respond very quickly. If the problem persists for more than 24 hours, or if you feel weakened or otherwise ill, consult your healthcare practitioner straight away.

Good Food

Simple foods that are full of natural goodness will provide you with the energy you need in order to function at your best and have ample amounts of available energy.

Good food is fresh, because the nutrients contained in the delicate cell walls of plants disintegrate quite quickly when exposed to air. This means that after ten days, although your courgette may look as well as it did when it came out of the ground, it will not be as nutritious, and you will not be receiving the vitamins and minerals you need from eating it. Some fruits and vegetables help us choose them while they are fresh, because they show visible signs of decay as they grow older. Others, like oranges, can be stored for months before they even begin to look the worse for wear. Many oranges are, in fact, stored for that long. They are often picked before they are ripe, and before the vitamins and micro-nutrients have had an opportunity to fully develop. Then they are packed, shipped and stored until they arrive on the shelves of your local shop or supermarket. Whatever vitamin C was present in their flesh at the beginning of their journey, there is precious little left after months in refrigerated storage.

The freshest food of all is that which you grow yourself, and this is an exciting way to monitor the quality of your food and ensure maximum nutrients. We can all grow something of our own, even if it is just mustard and cress on the windowsill, or sprouted beans on the draining board. Sprouted beans and seeds provide a real fillip for the system, being high in vegetable protein, Vitamin C, and other essential nutrients. Sprouting makes a dried or dead food come to life, and allows you to include a wide range of pulses in your diet. Sprouts rarely generate the same problems with intestinal gas that come from eating the cooked grain.

Choose from a variety of seeds, beans and grains, limiting one sort to each container. Use a sprouter if you have one, or otherwise place the damp pulses in a jar and cover with a sheet of kitchen paper. Rinse the contents three times a day with warm water, and watch the miracle of life unfurl in front of you. You will see the seeds crack and fresh, green spouts begin to grow within about two days. Harvest these after 3–5 days for the maximum benefits. You can add the sprouts to salads and sandwiches, or stir-fry them with other vegetables for a tasty and nutritious meal.

The following is a guide to some of the more common pulses, but do choose your own and begin to experiment.

Seed	Harvest after no. of days	Major benefits
Alfalfa	5-6	High Vitamin C
Chickpeas	4-6	Good protein source
Fenugreek	4-5	High mineral levels
Green lentils	3-5	Good protein source
Mung beans	2-5	Excellent pelvic cleanser
Soya beans	3-6	High protein and pre-hormone source
Sunflower seeds	4-6	Mineral mine

Good food is that which is able to provide you with all the nutrients you need from it, without being contaminated with toxins that will nullify its good effects. This means choosing naturally or organically grown foods over those which have been grown in a synthetic medium of assorted chemicals. Organic or naturally grown foods not only contain the elements we need to find in our food, but they also tend to look and taste better too. Perhaps most important of all is that they do *not* contain a complicated cocktail of artificial fertilisers, growth enhancers, fungicide treatments, pesticides, herbicides, bleaches and other chemicals, and are not subjected to the range of chemical processes — these days even apples are waxed with a petroleum-based substance.

Eczema is characterised by an intense itching and inflammation of the skin. It is strongly linked with food intolerance and will often respond well to changes in the diet, and to a blood-cleansing regime. Suspect foods include wheat, sugar, coffee, tea, chocolate, red meat, alcohol, dairy products, citrus fruits, nuts, seeds and tomatoes. Consider eliminating some of these foods from your diet for one month at a time, and see whether there is any response. Take additional oats, fatty fish, fruits and vegetables to supplement the diet, and a zinc or EFA supplement for three weeks. A daily cup of nettle tea will help cleanse the blood.

The growing number of allergies and health problems that we face as a society moves some to posit a direct link to the unknown effects of these chemical mixtures in our systems. Their cumulative effect, along with the consequences of air-borne pollutants, is to poison ourselves from the inside, as well as from the outside. Additionally, much of our nutritional good efforts can be wasted. When most of the goodies in a fruit or vegetable lie in or immediately below the skin, and this is the part we must remove in order to avoid the highest levels of contaminants, we are cheating ourselves out of valuable nutrients.

Choose fresh, naturally grown produce whenever you can. The financial cost is dropping all the time, and these foods are now much more freely available, and are present in much greater variety than they were, so every shopping list can include at least a few items. Once you have experienced the taste, the lack of waste and the health benefits that come from eating naturally grown foods, you will want to explore this market further.

If you are just starting out, consider the following foods to experiment with — they deliver the maximum difference in terms of taste and effects on the system (remember to include your favourite fruit and vegetable):

- apples
- carrots
- potatoes
- lemons
- lettuce
- grapes

Good food is also easy for the body to recognise, process and digest. This means that it is as close to its original form as possible, and not genetically altered, chemically copied, synthesised or adulterated. Genetically altered corn, soya and tomatoes have been the first to appear on the market, and although you would think these might be easy to spot, and therefore to avoid, they will tend to appear in any number of places courtesy of food processing methods.

> Corn is added to some potato crisps in the flavour dusting, forms part of the pastry in a number of bought cakes, puddings and biscuits, and appears in some composite meat products (sausages and pies), creamed soups, muesli and gravy mixes, ice creams, yoghurts, jams, beer, whiskey, glucose and cough syrups.

Altering the constitution of a food by processing and adulterating it with chemical taste enhancers, additives, life-extensors, preservatives and flavourings only serves to make manufacture easier. It rarely does anything for the food itself, and almost never enhances our health as consumers. As a general guideline, if you cannot pronounce or recognise the ingredient, or if it doesn't even have a name, just a number, then consider passing. Choose an alternative food that is more likely to do you good and provide the nutrients that you need. Do not be fooled by phrases such as 'nature-compatible' or 'nature-identical'. These are test-tube products that are no more natural than the building from which they came.

Whenever something has been added to the food or the process, it is often there because something necessary has been removed, or to compensate for a lack of nutrients. Vitamin enriched breads, for example, often contain the B-Complex because the outer husk of the grain, which is the original source of the B vitamins, has been removed. Other foods may be 'vitamin enriched'; that means that the chemical substitute for the vitamin has been added to the food, and this is usually to make up for the food having been denatured in some way. White bread often has vitamins added to it, because although these are present in wheat, they are removed with the husk when the flour is refined and bleached.

Soya flour is often used as a substitute or extender in the manufacture of bread, rolls, cakes and pastries. It is also present in soy sauce and a range of condiments, hard sweets, snacks, luncheon meats and burgers. It also appears in processed foods like pies, soups and ice-creams. Margarine and butter substitutes will also often contain soya.

Eating food as close to its natural condition as possible also means taking care with food preparation and cooking methods. When you slice into a vegetable and then wash it, you wash away a lot of the goodness. Similarly when you boil a vegetable and then strain it, much of the nutrients are poured down the sink.

- Eat some food in its raw state every day. Dress your salads inventively to maintain your interest.
- Prepare food carefully, washing before cutting it, and eating as soon after preparation as possible.
- Only peel fruit and vegetables when you have to, i.e. when the skin is inedible, or when the produce has not been naturally or organically grown.
- Steam rather than boil foods, and bake, grill, poach or stir-fry in minimal oil. These cooking methods will all help preserve nutrient levels.
- Retain cooking liquid to eat with the meal, or use as a base for sauce or soup.

The exception to this rule is food that is dried, especially fruit, which can add a valuable variety and range of nutrients to the diet. A 4 oz portion of dried apricots provides a day's potassium needs and a healthy dose of iron. Dried figs are a valuable source of calcium, very important for women, and are rich in magnesium, essential for healthy muscle activity. Raisins are excellent for enhancing elimination while maintaining energy levels, and are a good source of minerals. Nuts and seeds are also powerful additives to the diet, bringing a source of variety and an excellent range of minerals and micro-nutrients. They are also high in roughage, and therefore important to intestinal health. Drying is a useful way to store grains, fruits, vegetables and herbs, which can all be harvested when at their best and safely kept until they are needed.

Our need to be well-informed consumers is vital, because of the enormous influence food has on our ongoing and immediate health and well-being. If you were offered a piece of protein to eat that was full of the toxins and metabolic by-products of 18 months of a life that had been filled with no exercise and little pleasure, you might think twice about it. If you then found out this was from an animal who had been force-fed a range of artificial growth-enhancers, antibiotics and other pharmaceutical drugs, you would be wise to turn it down. If next you discover that this protein is full of the animal's hormones like the adrenaline which flooded its system because of the terrible pain and fear it had experienced during its final hours of life, you would be mad to eat it. This is the choice people make when they eat animals that have not been organically reared and humanely killed. Quite apart from the moral question, the effects on health can be devastating. From a moral standpoint, the way we tend to manufacture the animals that are in our care is indefensible. Many of us choose to eat animal protein, and for some of us this is a good and wise choice. It can only be that, however, when that meat is 'clean'.

What you eat is important, and so too is where you eat, with whom, when, how much, what it looks like, and how much you have. The smell of food has been shown to have as strong an effect on the body as actually eating it — so next time you breathe deeply of the aroma of fresh coffee, know that your body is responding in a very positive way, and you may not even need to go ahead and drink the cup to feel its positive effects. We know that taste is important to us, but rarely realise how strong our response is to the flavour of foods. Remember what it is like to bite on a slice of lemon — how it can make your toes curl and your eyes pucker up — that astringent effect can be felt throughout the body and has a marked effect on your digestive system, encourages your gall bladder to deal more effectively with the fats and oils that you eat, and stimulates a chain of beneficial reactions. How different this reaction is to the spreading warmth and satisfaction that comes from tasting something sweet like a milky drink. There is a role to be played by every taste-reaction, from the appetite-enhancing bitterness of salad leaves to the sour stomach-cleanser of salted or pickled foods. Include as wide a range of tastes and flavours in your meals to stimulate and encourage these effects, and to make your diet as rich and beneficial as possible.

The eight different tastes:

- Sour — vinegar
- Salty — sea water and seaweeds, celery and some other root vegetables

- Bitter — salad leaves, cumin, lemon rind, tonic water, turmeric, fenugreek
- Hot — chillis
- Pungent — mustard, onions and garlic, ginger, horseradish
- Putrid — hard cheeses, fermented foods like yoghurt and miso, and tofu
- Astringent — raw broccoli, avocado, lentils, peas and beans
- Sweet — sugar, honey, molasses, maple syrup

Food is a rather complex issue, and it is hard to separate it from our emotions and feelings and all our issues around being nurtured and loved. Perhaps the most important gift you can give yourself is to enjoy your mealtimes. Eating all the salad in the world will not do you good if you hate every mouthful. Although I would not advocate slavishly following your taste buds, especially if they have been under pressure and are likely to lead you towards processed, deep-fried, or sugary foods, a little of what you fancy can do you good. It is important to achieve balance in the whole matter of food and nourishment, just as it is in every other area of life. There is no place for obsession in good nourishment, so adopt as many of these simple guidelines as you are able to, and relax and enjoy your food.

Eating with the Seasons

Eating naturally makes sense — when you choose foods that are locally grown you are going to be eating what is in harmony with your body. Nature tends to provide us with the goodness that we need throughout the year, varying it through the seasons. During the winter months we have the stored energy of root vegetables and the grains saved from the autumn. spring brings with it a range of new sprouts. Summer provides us with an abundance of salad vegetables, fruits and berries, and autumn brings the harvest.

An occasional dish of strawberries can add something delightfully different to winter meals, but truly the food that you will benefit most from, and naturally be inclined towards, is that which is nourishing and warming. Long, slow-cooked meals and the roots that store all their energy in the ground are two valuable sources of additional energy for us during the colder months. Similarly, a Christmas pudding makes a treat of a dessert in the warmer weather, but summer tends to inspire us to enjoy the salad meals and rich abundance of berries and fruits that are growing then.

Cooking methods go hand in hand with the foods that are available naturally. Long slow cooking like baking and oven roasting suit the greater energy requirements of the colder months, while quick, spring-type energy is perfectly catered for in stir-frying and brief steaming.

Herbs and Spices

These are an essential part of every healthy diet. Their effects range from the immediate change they can cause in our appreciation of a meal by enhancing the aroma and the scent, to the marked benefits on a medicinal level. Often the distinguishing line between herbs and vegetables is blurred, and many people eat spring greens containing dandelion leaves and young nettles, for example. All herbs and spices, being plants, store valuable nutrients and are able to yield these when we take them in our food. They also form the basis of many of our medicines and herbal remedies.

> Herbs and spices used in cooking almost always have medicinal effects. The caraway, cardamom and fennel seeds found in curry and spice mixes all encourage the digestion and help prevent flatulence. Chew a handful of these seeds after eating if you suffer with abdominal gas.

Some common herbs and spices are shown below with their nutritional and curative values, and it is worth experimenting to find those that suit you best.

Herb/Spice	Actions and properties
Bay	Warming, an excellent digestive aid. Add to any cooked meals.
Black pepper	Warming, a good digestive aid but may irritate the bowel, so use judiciously.
Cardamom	Calms the system and stimulates digestion. Excellent in sweets and dairy puddings and to flavour hot water for drinking. Said to benefit the reproductive organs and increase fertility.

Herb/Spice	Actions and properties
Coriander or Cilantro	Cools the digestive system, relieves the urinary tract, and helps eliminate gas from the system. Grows esily on a windowsill, or outdoors during the summer. Chop and add to salads and stir fries or as a garnish on any meal.
Dandelion	Promotes the elimination of excess fluid from the system.
Fennel	Cools the system, sweetens the breath and settles the stomach.
Horseradish	Opens the lungs and clears the nasal passages. High in Vitamin C.
Juniper	Traditionally used to flavour gin, so their taste will be familiar. These berries are a powerful and warming diuretic, and useful whenever there is bladder infection and to strengthen the kidneys. Crush and add to any cooked meal.
Parsley	A good source of iron and other minerals, high in Vitamin C.
Sage	A wonderful remedy for the neck and throat, and for use as a gargle. Relieves excessive sweating and will help stop the flow of breast milk, Grows easily and rewards with beautiful long, spiked flower heads. Use the leaves and add to all baked meals, and chop in salads.

Herb/Spice	Actions and properties
Thyme	An excellent cleansing herb, suitable for use in all inhalants, and to burn to rid the home of germs from the sick room. It has excellent aromatic value and can be added to salads, soups, and all cooked meals. Especially useful when cooking meat.
Turmeric	Aids protein digestion, a powerful wound healer.

Keeping a Diet Diary

This is an excellent way to focus on what you are really eating and how you feel about your food, as well as showing you how your body responds, and what patterns exist in your current diet. Aim to record everything that you eat and drink in your diary, at the time that you consume it. You will need to include as much information as possible, including who you were with when you ate, whether the meal was home-cooked or shop bought, etc., and whether you were feeling relaxed or tense immediately prior to the meal.

Keep your diary for at least a week, and longer if possible. Try not to do anything other than record your food habits, leaving your analysis until the end of the week. Then you will be able to pick out any trends, or food groups that seem important. Look for your eating habits, and then for your favourite foods and ways of eating. Then see if there is any connection with how you feel emotionally and physically, and what, when or how you ate.

Use this daily page as a guide to formatting your own personalised diary.

Date			
Season		Weather	
	Time	Food	Drinks
Breakfast			
Snacks			
Lunch			
Tea			
Supper			
Bedtime			
Feelings after eating:			
Feelings at end of day:			
Energy levels:			
Additional Notes:			

Food Allergies

Whenever there is an over-dependence on any type of food in our diet, there is a risk that the body may at some time begin to reject it. This can sometimes be seen generationally, with, for example, people of Mediterranean descent exhibiting allergic responses to olives or onions, both staples within their traditional diet.

> Sufferers from migraines may discover that food allergies play a strong part in the pattern of these painful and debilitating headaches. Chocolate, strong cheeses, cured meats and red wine are among the common food triggers, but there may be negative responses to foods as diverse as peppers and avocados. Avoid these main triggers if you have a problem with migraines, and look to the ways you can manage the stress in your life. Keeping a diet diary will help you identify other food triggers that are unique to you.

Keeping a diet diary is a good way to begin to discover whether there are any foods that trouble you. This is all an allergy is. In some people it can cause a definite and instant reaction — such as those whose mouth and throat begin to swell up within moments of eating a peanut — although these life-threatening responses are extremely rare. More often, the symptoms of food allergy are cumulative and subtly debilitating, making them harder to identify.

Common allergic reactions include:

- low energy levels
- headaches
- fatigue
- abdominal pain and bloating
- forgetfulness
- eczema
- cold or flu-type symptoms
- lip, mouth and tongue blisters
- depression
- digestive complaints (diarrhoea, constipation, indigestion)
- weight-gain and/or loss outside your normal range
- mood changes

An amazing number of people show signs of wheat and dairy allergies. This can often be because of our over-dependence on them in our usual diet. Consider when you last ate wheat, and you might need to stop and think for a moment, but it was in the toast you may have had at breakfast, the mid-morning pastry, the sandwich for lunch, the afternoon cake and the pasta dinner. Cow's dairy products appear in much the same way, squeezing their way into all sorts of unexpected places. As well as the milk you pour on your cereal and add to your tea and coffee, they include the butter on your bread, the cheese in your sandwich and on your pasta and the white sauce on your vegetables. They also appear in most prepared puddings and desserts.

> Wheat proteins have been found in over 60 per cent of arthritic joints. If you suspect that wheat might be causing a problem for you, or if you experience arthritic pain and joint changes and want to try eliminating wheat, do so for at least one month. Prepare carefully so that you will not be tempted to have any wheat at all, but will have substitutes and alternatives already in place. Symptoms of arthritis respond very well to naturopathic dietary therapy.

Eliminating a suspected allergen from your diet means becoming vigilant about reading the labels of everything you eat to ensure that you are truly eliminating something from your diet. To do this effectively, decide to avoid the food or substance for a period of one month, and keep a diet diary throughout this time, especially to chart the balance of your new diet and to note the health changes you are experiencing. Do not choose to exclude more than one major food group at a time, and do make sure that your diet is providing you with alternative sources of nutrients or energy. It is recommended that you consult your healthcare adviser for support and information if you feel that you would respond well to significant dietary changes.

Consider making some basic changes to your diet if you are overly reliant on any particular food, or if your diet is rich in foods that you know are not health-enhancing. These might include stimulants such as caffeine, foods high in saturated fats, wheat and cow's dairy produce.

The following substitution table suggests some alternatives to consider for those wishing to exclude a particular food, and also finds some everyday options that can be used to widen your diet, or to help replace foods on which you are reliant.

Food	Replace with:
Caffeine (present in coffee, tea, colas, chocolate, some pain-killers, etc.)	Herbal teas. Dilute fruit and vegetable juices
Tannin in tea	Water, grain-based coffee substitutes, Barleycup
Red meat	Fish and seafood, chicken and poultry, soya beans and tofu
Cow's dairy milk and milk products	Goat's and sheep's milk, cheese and yoghurts, soya, rice and nut milks and cheeses
Wheat	Other grains such as rye, buckwheat, amaranth barley, soya, rice, etc. — all can be found as flours, pastas, breads, cakes, etc.
Bread	Rice-cakes, rye crackers, corn tortillas, oat cakes
Salt	Gomasio (sesame seed and salt mix), herbs and spices
MSG and artificial flavour enhancers	Nature's own flavour enhancers — herbs and spices

There is a strong connection between cow's dairy foods and sinus congestion. Giving up cow's dairy foods can mean an end to stubborn sinus complaints and resultant problems with headaches, colds and nasal congestion. Goat's milk and sheep's milk are readily available substitutes which may well be easier on the body, and many grains can also yield a 'milk', thus providing a liquid and all the associated nutrients, e.g. soya milk is a rich alternative source of protein, and rice milk is high in calcium.

Fasting — When Not to Eat

Sometimes the best thing you can do for your body is not to eat. Fasting is something that we all tend to do quite naturally. Most children will follow their instincts and ignore food altogether on occasion, or if they are feeling at all ill or under the weather. Digestion requires a great deal of energy, and it is wonderful to give the body a holiday from that work so that it can return to the task refreshed and revitalised. This also gives the body an opportunity to divert its resources to other areas that might be in need of attention. This is what happens when your appetite disappears just as soon as you develop a fever, or come down with a virus — your body is needing to do some hard work and needs all its available resources. Fasting when you are not feeling ill at all is like a gift to the body. It gives your whole system a chance to catch up with any backlog or housekeeping chores, and leaves you feeling refreshed and re-energised.

Fasting can take many forms — it is not at all scary, and can be quite delicious. A modified fast can take the form of eating all your favourite fruits for a day or longer, or simply drinking juices or fortified juices throughout the day. The type of fast you choose to follow will depend upon your reasons for doing this, your basic state of health, and whether you have ever followed a fast before.

> Bad breath is almost always a sign that all is not well in part of the system — either within the gut or in the mouth. Fasting is an excellent way to allow the body to heal any minor imbalances, and will almost certainly resolve the complaint. Become vigilant and the symptom can help you to identify dietary excesses and the early stages of ill-health. Chew a handful of fresh parsley for an immediate breath-cleanser that is especially useful to freshen the mouth after eating garlic. It also delivers a good dose of Vitamin C to the mouth and will help with any localised problem.

If you have never done this before, and you are basically quite healthy, then a lovely choice is to eat fruit for a day. This is a simple fillip for the digestion, maintains your energy levels, and introduces your conscious mind, and your body, to the notion of fasting. Do this during the spring or summer months, when the range and variety of fruits is at its most appealing, and when your body is most receptive to following a varied fruit day. Prepare for this by planning ahead. Make sure you buy in a good selection of fruits that you like, and plan a day when you do not have to meet too many commitments. This should be seen as a gift to yourself, and can tie in wonderfully with any other treats you may want to enjoy.

The basic rules for fasting are the same whether you are spending a day eating mixed fruits or are following a water-only fast:

- Always let your health adviser or natural healthcare practitioner know what you are doing.
- Monitor your fast carefully, taking note of any strong physical, emotional or energy changes that take place.
- Make sure that you drink at least one glass of water every 1½ hours.
- Never fast for more than three days without the guidance and monitoring of your healthcare practitioner.

Monitoring the changes that you experience whilst you are fasting will give you a wonderful insight into the health priorities that your body is dealing with. It also serves to connect you with what you are doing in a tremendously useful way. Learn to take your pulse, and record the readings when you wake up in the morning, then every three hours or so until you go to bed. You can also take your temperature, look at the state of your eyes and your tongue, and check the quality of your breath. You will soon recognise your own individual pattern of health changes that occur when you are fasting. Usually these are signs that your body is eliminating toxins from your system, and the most noticeable of these is in the clarity of the whites of your eyes, and the degree of coating you will see on your tongue.

Pulse rates and basic temperature will vary through the day, depending on how active you are and how much work the body is doing.

If you have established regular fruit fasts into your routine, or if you have a strong constitution and wish to try the next stage, consider spending a day taking only juices and water. This rests the digestive system substantially, while continuing to provide a range of nutritional and tasty drinks to meet ongoing energy requirements. Choose from a range of vegetables and fruits, and if possible make sure that you juice them yourself for maximum benefit. A mixed juice day comprising any and all of the vegetables and fruits that you enjoy will be a treat for your system, and a pleasure for your taste-buds. Refine this further by choosing only one fruit or vegetable. In terms of improving elimination from your system, some choices will be faster or more effective than others. Let your tastes guide you, or choose from some in the following table:

Choice of Food	Special Benefits
Apricots	Rich source of Vitamin A, iron and other minerals. Prevent constipation.
Pineapple	Wonderfully eliminative, especially for meat eaters. The enzymes in the pineapple will aid digestion and break down any accumulations in the digestive tract.

Choice of Food	Special Benefits
Beetroot	An excellent liver tonic, useful for those who drink alcohol, or who experience any difficulty digesting fats.
Apple	Strongly soothing for the stomach and the entire digestive system. Useful in all chronic or long-standing conditions, and the perfect choice for autumn and spring cleanses.
Carrot	A good source of Vitamin A, and useful for the respiratory system. A protective agent against colds and flu, it will also help brighten the eyes. Warming, and an excellent choice when re-introducing foods after a water fast.
Grape	Wonderful blood-sugar balancer, and strong blood cleanser. A good year-round choice for maintaining energy levels and achieving maximum benefits.
Lettuce	Will help rid the body of bloating, while soothing and calming the nerves. Excellent source of chlorophyll and a good blood oxygenator that will increase energy levels and speed the rate of healing.
Grapefruit	Excellent for reducing fevers, and for all gall-bladder insufficiency, or when gall-stones are present. Alternate with pineapple for maximum benefits.

Only when your system is used to regular fasting, and you are experiencing the positive benefits of it, should you consider following a plain water fast. This is an amazingly healing thing to do, and will be the treatment of choice for many ongoing and acute health concerns. It is always best to follow a fast such as this with the monitoring and guidance of an experienced natural healthcare practitioner. Never follow any type of fast for more than three days without such assistance.

Whatever type of fast you choose, the following guidelines are important to your success:

- Make sure that you drink enough water, even though you may not be feeling thirsty. Drink this hot if you are feeling cold.
- Take some exercise — as much as you can manage.
- Allow yourself extra time to complete tasks — your energy levels may fluctuate.
- Take regular rests — nap if you feel inclined, otherwise simply rest.
- Be as flexible as possible. You may notice many changes in all your basic patterns, from toilet habits to sleep requirements.
- Make notes of all the changes, symptoms, and experiences that occur throughout your fast.

Every fast has three distinct stages: Before, During and Afterwards, and each is of equal importance.

Before you fast

Plan ahead in terms of making sure you have shopped for the things you will need, and have thought it through adequately. Endeavour to choose a time when you will not be in difficult situations of any type, whether emotionally or socially, or when there is too great a work load. Prepare for your fast by eating simply the day before, and remembering to drink lots.

After you fast

This is a crucial time for building on the good work you will have accomplished during the fast, and it is a time to take things simply, making it easy on your body to switch from one type of work to another. Plan the reintroduction of foods carefully, taking things slowly, and always imagining yourself having eaten the food first. Close your eyes, and see how it feels to imagine the food in your stomach. If you have been juicing, make your first meal a piece of the fruit or vegetable that you have juiced, so follow an apple juice fast with a whole apple, and then about two hours later, eat another apple with something else, perhaps a carrot or a pear. Move towards cooked foods, and a mixture of different foods, very slowly, paying attention to how you feel the whole time. Remember to drink lots.

What to Drink

Water is a wonderful drink for the whole body. It is thirst-quenching and provides an excellent medium for the body to eliminate all water-soluble toxins. We need to drink about 2 litres of water every day in order to stay well hydrated, and to achieve optimum kidney function. Drinking water has a marked calming effect on the stomach, and will often soothe an irritable stomach or one that is over-hungry. Often hunger can be mistaken for a desire to drink, and taking two glasses of water will appease and settle the stomach.

The things we tend to add to water can have marked effects in the system. Caffeine is a strong stimulant, and although some digestions seem to be heightened by the acidity of the drink, it is worthy of respect for the drug that it is. Taking several cups of coffee every day makes you a drug addict. If you stop straight away, the withdrawal symptoms can be mildly unpleasant. Usually they will extend to headaches and a general feeling of lack of energy and lethargy — all the things to make you want to get another hit. Tea also contains caffeine and tannin, another strong acting substance. Treat these two drinks as the medicine that they can be — useful when you need to benefit from their effects, but certainly not something to add to your basic intake.

Investigate the range of fruit, vegetable and herbal teas to add variety and provide a tasty hot drink. There is also an excellent variety of grain drinks to substitute for coffee, ranging from those made from mixed grains to specialist drinks like Barleycup. Consider drinking boiled water first thing in the morning, and a little while after meals, to aid digestion. This is a very soothing and pleasant drink on its own, or add a few cardamom pods, a slice of lemon or some fennel seeds to vary the taste.

Herbal Tea	Additional Benefits
Camomile	Calming and relaxing, soothes the digestion and de-stresses the system.
Hawthorn	Excellent for toning the heart muscle and a tonic for the cardio-vascular system.
Lemon balm	Refreshing and soothing, seems to impart some of the flavour of summer, and lifts spirits.
Nettle	Good blood-cleanser and high in minerals. An excellent seasonal choice during the spring.
Peppermint	Aromatic and fragrant, has a cooling effect on the system and will aid digestion.
Rosehip	Rich source of Vitamin C.

Juices are a valuable source of neutral fluid and contain all the nutrients of the fruit or vegetable. Freshly squeezed or extracted juices will contain the highest concentration of Vitamin C, and will also taste best. Dilute all juices 50/50 with water to heighten their uptake in the body and increase fluid levels.

Always take care to ensure the purity and quality of everything you drink and eat. Attention to this will provide you with the best possible inner environment for continued good health. It is also a wonderfully healing thing to care so well for yourself, and to want and deliver only the best on such a vital level of your existence. Our bodies work so hard to enable us to continue doing all that we choose and need to, and making every mealtime a loving communion with ourselves is an act of gratitude to the Creator.

Chapter 4

ENERGY, MOVEMENT AND HEALING

The way your body is, whether you are moving it or not, is vitally important to your health. The tone of the muscles, the position of the joints and the freedom of the vertebrae are all keys to a well-functioning body. The spine itself is at the hub of a whole range of physical activities like breathing, digestion and elimination, and that is before you even begin to move.

The nervous system carries information to and from the tissues. This is how the impulse to move or to function is relayed to an organ or a muscle, and is the same system by which messages from the tissues, like their position, or pain, reach the brain. The individual nerves which run to each part of the body are protected by the bones of the spine as they travel down your body. They leave that bony protection at different levels, and it is imperative that this site of departure is unhindered. Any spinal misalignment, or even muscle tension and poor posture, can all occlude this vital area, and mean that less than perfect information is able to get through to the body. When this occurs, it also means that the brain is receiving less than perfect information about how each area is functioning and what its needs are.

Nature has designed the body to work pretty well as it is. When we rearrange its positioning, for instance by spending hours every day in a posture that does not suit us, we do not allow the body to work at an optimum. This can mean that functions like breathing and digestion, the breakdown of fats and movement of tissues can all be adversely affected. Witness this for yourself next time you spend an evening sitting slumped forward in an armchair — notice how your breathing is necessarily more shallow, and how common it is to feel some degree of indigestion. Sitting in an upright position for an hour after eating will often resolve any minor digestive concerns.

Taking care of our bodies means looking at a whole range of positions in which we place ourselves, from our seating to our choice of bed. How you sit, on what, and for how long have more of an impact on your body than the actions that you take once you begin to move. In much the same way, the longest time that you are likely to spend at rest in any one place is in bed every night, and an inappropriate mattress can make a world of difference to how your body works. A good, supportive mattress will allow your heavier areas around your shoulders and hips to sink into it, and still support the rest of your body without too much 'give'. Rearranging the position you choose to sleep in can do a lot to resolve ongoing aches and pains. Keeping a pillow down in the bed for you to place under your knees if you lie on your back, or between your knees while you are on your side, will help relieve any stress on your lower back, and ease the position of your neck. Not using too many pillows, and making sure that you are not in a draught, are the other two most important factors.

One of the most common causes of neck pain is a problem in the lower back. When we put on weight, and the bowel is sluggish, then the pull forward on the lower back can be immense. Add to this the mechanical effects of wearing high heels, and the increase in the natural curve of the lower back can be phenomenal. Whatever happens there is reflected in the neck region, where the bones are smaller and lighter, and more prone to being misplaced. Tightening the abdominal muscles, and releasing the lower back will usually allow the neck to release and sort out the cause of the problem. Understanding the need to remedy the physical problem and learn new postures goes a long way towards a cure. Neck problems are more common in larger-breasted women, whose need for good posture is increased in order to counteract the forward pull on the chest wall.

Good posture simply means using your body in the way it was designed to work best. This means making the most of your body's capabilities, and not abusing its ability to adapt. The most important aspect of good posture is not how you move, but the positions you hold when you are still. This is when the muscles that you use for movement and work are not in use, and any potential strain is placed directly on your joints. Your spine has its own natural curves; one forward curve in the neck, a slightly rounded, backward curve in the shoulder region, and another forward curve in your low back. Your centre of gravity depends on the integrity of this line, and the sweeping curves make sure that your whole body stays in balance.

Imagine, then, shifting your whole centre of gravity so that you are in fact leaning forward and taking all your weight on your toes. The gentle sweeping curves of your spine automatically realign and try to cope with this position. Women who wear high heels place this type of stress on their spine for hours and hours every day. Add to this the effect of suspending a heavy weight from one shoulder, which drags one side of the body down and means that all symmetry in that plane is also lost. This is the effect of carrying a heavy shoulder-bag.

Simply switching to a lower or flat heel, and not wearing a bag on one shoulder can relieve tremendous stress in your back and feet, and will have a positive effect not just on any aches and pains but also on your energy levels, breathing pattern and digestion. Many bunions, corns and other foot problems are caused by a combination of ill-fitting shoes and the fact that the shoes have heel heights that are not appropriate for us. Try this simple experiment to see whether your shoes are a good fit for you: Stand in your bare foot on a piece of paper and draw around it using a thick pen. Now stand in your shoe on another piece of paper, and draw around that using a thick pen. There is often little comparison between the natural shape of your foot and the shoe in which you house it for up to eighteen hours a day.

Choosing shoes that fit the shape of your foot can have a positive effect on corns, fallen arches, bunions and other foot problems. Take off your shoes and stockings or socks and allow your feet to breathe for as long as you can every day. Encourage your toes back into their natural alignment by packing the spaces in between them with cotton wool pads, and by working the small postural muscles in the foot: practise picking up objects, turning pages of a magazine or paper and holding a pen and drawing with your toes.

Work those muscles further by walking barefoot on a range of different surfaces — especially those with some 'give' like sand and earth.

Various natural specialities focus on working with posture and movement. These include the Alexander Technique and the Feldenkrais Method. You can start to notice your own posture right now, and see how you really feel.

Take a moment to close your eyes and scan quickly through your body, noting where you feel any areas of tension or discomfort. Just let your attention wander from your head right down to your toes, including as much of your body as you can along the way. The classic places to hold tension are in the forehead and jaw, the neck and shoulders, the stomach, low back and bottom. Some people hold their toes all scrunched up, or their chins. You may find any spot that feels tight and could be uncomfortable. Sometimes you will notice it as being down one side of your body, or there may be several points that feel tense.

If you repeat this body scan in an hour's time, and again an hour after that, you are likely to find that the same places are tense. One of the simplest and most immediate ways to relax is to take a deep breath, and imagine you are breathing right into the centre of the spot that is tight, and then having refreshed it, allow it to relax again as you breathe out.

Relaxation is an art form in itself, and there are many different ways to achieve this. For some who hold tension in their bodies, it is necessary to use that pent-up energy in a physical way, so going for a brisk walk or undertaking any kind of activity will do the job. Others will find that their minds don't seem to stop, and that causes tension. Here the remedy needs to be in finding a way to allay mental anxiety and concerns, and list-making is a wonderful way to do that. Making sure that you have a pencil and paper always to hand means that all those thoughts can be recorded, and reduces the need to hold the memory in your mind. With time, this method can be wonderfully successful. Everybody responds to an inner message that says that all is well, you are safe and can now relax. Try this for yourself:

Find somewhere to be relaxed and undisturbed. Close your eyes and make sure you are sitting comfortably. Start to scan your body just as you did before, starting at the top of your head. Be aware of your breathing, and with every out-breath, say the word 'relax' to yourself silently. Whenever you reach a part of your body that feels tense or uncomfortable, keep breathing, and rest your attention there for a while. Say silently to yourself: 'I am safe and secure in my own energy, and am now able to relax.' Repeat this until you start to feel better in that spot, and continue on down your body until you reach your toes.

This is a great exercise to do in bed at night if you are unable to sleep.

A good posture is one that works for you and allows your body to be comfortable and effective. It is always relaxed. The old-fashioned army-type shoulders back, chest out rigidity doesn't actually work for most people. What tends to happen as we tense is the body becomes shorter and hunched together. The following exercises will gently lengthen the body, and can be practised whenever you think of them. Do them regularly for best effect:

- Imagine that attached to the back of your head is a long, thin, artist's paintbrush reaching up as an extension of your spine. Allow your neck to lengthen so that the hairs of the brush are able to gently dust the ceiling.
- Picture a piece of strong, fine silken cord attached to the front of the bone in the middle of your chest. See the other end attaching to a hook set into the ceiling right above your head. Allow the cord to tighten and gently lift your ribs and your whole trunk. Feel your chin fall back slightly as your chest rises, and any tension in the back of your neck disappears. Keep the silk taut.
- When standing, bend your knees slightly so that your weight drops down and the hollow of your back disappears. At the same time tighten your lower abdominal muscles to further flatten out that hollow.

Back pain is sometimes caused by remaining fixed in one position for too long. This is especially so if you need to stand in one place for any length of time. Shift your weight from one foot to another, and bend your knees slightly so that your thigh muscles, rather than the ligaments in your spine, are doing the work of holding you up. Work to tighten your abdominal muscles so that they will form a natural girdle to protect your back. Keep your breathing deep and relaxed, so that your whole body is moving as much as it can. Rotate your head on your neck, and relax your shoulders to relieve secondary points of tension. Once you are able to move freely again, make some gentle stretches and a few expansive movements with your arms to open up your trunk, free your breathing and mobilise your spine.

Movement

Having developed an easy, relaxed, resting posture, you will find that the way you move is changed. Your body should be feeling more open and agile, so build on the good work of your resting posture, and make sure that you use your body to best effect. Altering the way you move means that you can protect areas that have been under stress, and develop the muscle groups that you need in order for your body to work best.

We need to move regularly in order to stay alive! The condition of our muscles depends upon some regular use, and our metabolism responds to general activity. The continued presence of substances, e.g. hormones, that we need in order to stay well is dependent upon motion, and the way that our food is moved through the gut is hastened and improved by the gentle squeezing and stretching that occurs when we walk. Besides anything else, we usually feel better when we are able to move and stretch and feel our body in motion.

Beyond the need for regular exercise to improve the capability of all our muscles, including the heart, exercise does a lot to elevate the mood, put a spring in the step, bring a glow to the skin, and generally make one look and feel better. Finding an exercise you like has never been easier. We tend to think of good exercise as being centred around aerobic activity. Although we need to be stretched aerobically, this can happen in a multitude of ways and a variety of places, from the dance-floor to the bedroom — it doesn't always have to be in an aerobics class. Anything that makes your heart beat faster, and your breathing become fuller, is good news on the exercise front. If you enjoy walking, and notice this effect after striding out, then that is fine. If cycling is more to your taste, or dancing, or running, or working out in a gym, then that is just great too. If you enjoy what you are doing, you are likely to continue doing it, and life is too short to spend your time doing things you hate.

Walking is one of the best all-round exercises you can take. It involves the whole body in a rhythmic, easy movement that benefits every part of you. It automatically gets you outdoors, and in theory at least ensures you are getting some fresh air. Make sure you walk where it is as unpolluted as possible, and where the surface is best — concrete paving slabs can cause problems for the joints, so choose grass, tarmacadam, sand, soil or gravel. Stride out when you walk, and keep your pace nice and brisk, swinging your arms a little to increase your aerobic capacity. Walking is especially beneficial for women, who need to ensure adequate weight-bearing activity to reduce the effects of the bone-thinning disease osteoporosis which can cause problems after the menopause.

Walking is one of the best practical cures for constipation. With each step, the gut is gently squeezed and stretched, and this encourages the mechanical action of the bowel. Hill climbing, and even walking on a small incline, will increase the effect, and regular walks should ensure good bowel health. Walking will also help keep the abdominal and waist muscles in shape.

Even when you do not consider yourself to be actively exercising, it can be very beneficial to look at the way you move and use your body. Many of us favour one hand over the other, but will find that we take this a lot further and actually use one side of our body much more than the other. Check this for yourself — what side of your desk is your telephone; what arm do you use to push the vacuum cleaner; which foot do you kick with; which arm do you use to pick things up and carry them?

Small adjustments to the way we do things can make a big difference to how easy we feel in our body. Choosing a better sitting position can take pressure off joints that were not designed to deal with it, and relieve sites of constant muscle tension. Walking more often and more freely can mobilise the entire body rather than risk compounding any structural difficulty. This can work to reduce digestive problems and encourage fuller breathing too. Moving your chair to a new place so that you change the angle at which you read or watch television can make a difference, as will putting the telephone to your other ear, making sure your feet are right underneath you when you move to get up, and a host of other minor adjustments. Experiment for yourself by first noting your physical habit patterns, and then giving yourself a rest from them for a while.

Sprains and strains will respond well to careful home treatment. Immediately you feel pain or discomfort:

- Stop what you are doing and rest the affected area. This will protect you.
- Apply some ice wrapped in a cloth or tea-towel, or anything else that is available from the freezer, such as a packet of frozen peas. This will help reduce any swelling and also have a pain-killing effect.
- Hold the ice in place by tying it around the area, or placing it within a sock or something similar. This will apply some pressure to the area and further reduce swelling.
- Raise the affected area above the level of your heart — for example, do not only lift your leg, but lie down while you do it. This will speed the rate of blood supply and healing.

Stretch Carefully

When we think of stretching, we think of reaching towards something, working outwards and extending ourselves. We think of putting in extra effort and exerting greater pull. When we stretch the body, we need to rethink our ideas and do it in a way that allows us to relax down into feeling the extent or full range of the area's own capability. Rather than seeing what we can push ourselves into and make ourselves do, we need to settle into discovering what we are already capable of. Each muscle has its own innate capacity for elongation and elegance, and when we gently, slowly stretch in a contained way, we simply allow that muscle to discover its own potential.

There are many different ways to stretch and tone your muscles. Slow, gentle stretches that include working with your breath will often be the most effective. Our knowledge of the gross anatomy of the body, combined with an appreciation for its subtler energetic channels, allows us to develop a personalised system of everyday exercise that will perfectly suit our own changing needs. Know where your large muscle groups are, pay attention to the smaller muscles, and approach exercise from a viewpoint of increasing health rather than minimising perceived figure faults. This will allow exercise to become part of a rejuvenating, re-energising plan for optimum health and well-being.

There are many different exercise systems that focus on this approach to lengthening the body and increasing energy levels through opening and releasing any deep muscle tensions. The added benefits of choosing this type of exercise are the wonderful sense of relaxation, and the relative safety if they are performed with care — there is little chance of dropping a weight or falling off a step. Yoga is perhaps the best known in the West, although the exercises themselves form only part of a much larger discipline that includes meditation, dietary care, breath-work and spiritual guidance. When practised well, yoga can be a very useful form of exercise, especially for those over 35 years of age, and anyone prone to stiffness or arthritis.

Gross anatomy tells us where everything is in our body in relation to everything else, and what it does. Subtler systems map the energy flow of the body and connect our emotions and feelings with what happens to us on a physical level. The Eastern energy maps provide us with a way of understanding the basics of what happens in our lives, and how this manifests itself physically.

These chart the movement of energy along lines or vessels called meridians. They run throughout the body, connecting deep structures like organs to the surface of the skin, and providing a means of communication. Yoga is among the several systems of medicine that use energy maps. These systems include traditional Chinese medicine, whose acupuncture maps are based on them, and the Japanese bodywork tradition of Shiatsu. You can work on these meridians yourself using a personalised system of Shiatsu called *Do-In*.

Do-In

This is a generalised work-out that carefully stimulates all the meridians and really wakes your body up. You can do this in the morning, or whenever you feel like being energised and refreshed. Start by standing comfortably with your feet flat on the floor, about shoulder-width apart, and your knees slightly bent. Take a deep breath, and relax any tension you feel in your back and throughout your body.

Form your hands into loose fists, and let your arms hang loosely by your sides. Allow your fists to gently hit against the outside of your thighs, keeping your wrists loose and your arms heavy and relaxed. The beating action of your hands needs to be very relaxed and gentle, using just the weight of your fists to make an impression. Once you are confident that your 'beating' is relaxed and easy, you are going to work your way all over your body, waking up your meridians and muscles.

Start at the top of your head, gently 'knocking' over your scalp and then down the back and sides of your neck with both your loose fists. Continue down each arm in turn, taking lines down its length until you reach the hand; across and down the front of your chest, and over each shoulder. Wrap your arms around your body to reach your back, and work down your sides and your abdomen as well. 'Knock' your way around your hips, down the front, back, and sides of each leg, and then lifting one foot at a time, work over the sole of each foot.

Stand still for a moment or two after finishing to allow yourself to enjoy the feelings and sensations in your body after having given yourself this wonderful wake-up call.

Makka-Ho

The Japanese system of stretches called *Makka-Ho* works more specifically with the system of meridians or energy pathways through the body, gently stretching them and the muscles and joints through which they flow, and easing their passage. Each of the six stretches works on a pair of meridians, and they are best followed in sequence. Each stretch needs to be practised with careful breathing to achieve the maximum positive effect.

Try this exercise system for a month, and see how you feel. If any of the stretches or postures causes you pain or discomfort, stop immediately and consider consulting your naturopath, osteopath or chiropractor for a physical structural assessment.

Breathe out when moving into and out of each position. Hold each stretch for three deep breaths, and let yourself relax further into the stretch with each out-breath.

1. The Lungs and Large Intestine

Stand with your feet a little way apart, and your knees 'soft'. Link your thumbs behind your back, breathe in and gently extend your arms behind you. Keeping your thumbs linked together, breathe out, and bring your arms up over your head and let their weight pull them forwards in front of you. Allow yourself to bend to follow your arms, and keep your fingers straight. Stay in this position for three deep breaths, feeling the stretch as you relax further with each out-breath. Take another deep breath in, and as you breathe out, slowly straighten up, bringing your arms back to rest behind your back.

2. The Stomach and Spleen

Kneel on the floor and place your hands flat on the floor behind you. Take a deep breath in, and as you breathe out, raise your hips, and feel the stretch in the front of your legs. Keep your jaw relaxed, and let your mouth fall open a little. Let your head reach back a little, as you stretch the whole of the front of your body. Stay in this position for three deep breaths, feeling the stretch as you raise your hips a little further with each out-breath. Take another deep breath in, and as you breathe out, slowly lower your hips and return to the kneeling position.

3. The Heart and Small Intestine

Stay on the floor, and swing around so that you are sitting on it. Bend both your knees up, and let them fall gently out as you take a hold on your ankles. Keep your feet together and pull your toes in towards your body. Take a deep breath in, and as you breathe out, hold your toes, and curl your body forwards so that your elbows and knees stretch down to the floor. Stay in this position for three deep breaths, feeling the stretch as you relax further with each out-breath. Take another deep breath in, and as you breathe out, slowly straighten up into a sitting position.

4. The Kidneys and Bladder

Straighten out your legs so that they are lying directly out in front of you. Relax your feet. Take a deep breath in, and as you breathe out, stretch up, reaching towards the ceiling with both arms. Let the weight of your straight arms carry you forward as you bend down to bring your chest towards your knees. Keep your back straight, and feel the stretch all the way from the base of your spine up through your neck. Use your eyes to look forward and across the room. Stay in this position for three deep breaths, feeling the stretch as you relax a little further with each out-breath. Take another deep breath in, and as you breathe out, slowly straighten back up into a sitting position.

5. Heart Protector and Triple Heater

Cross your legs in front of you, or sit in the lotus or half lotus yoga position if you are able. Cross your arms over in front of you, and rest your right hand, palm upwards on your left knee, and your left hand, palm upwards on your right knee. Take a deep breath in, and as you breathe out, stretch forward, keeping your back straight, and aim your forehead towards the floor in front of you. Feel the stretch in your arms. Stay in this position for three deep breaths, feeling the stretch as you relax a little further with each out-breath. Take another deep breath in, and as you breathe out, slowly straighten back up into a sitting position, then uncross your arms, and then your legs.

6. The Liver and Gall Bladder

Open your legs so that they are straight, and pointing out to the sides as far apart as you can comfortably keep them. Hold the left side of your waist with your right hand, and reach up towards the ceiling with your left hand. Take a deep breath in, and as you breathe out, allow the weight of your left hand to carry you down to your right, aiming your right ear towards your right knee. Feel the stretch in the side of your body and your legs. Stay in this position for three deep breaths, feeling the stretch as you relax a little further with each out-breath. Take another deep breath in, and as you breathe out, slowly straighten back up into a sitting position. Take a deep breath in, and release it. Then begin again, stretching to the other side.

After completing all the exercises, your body should feel pleasantly sparkling and alive, and you will normally feel as though you have lots of energy. You may find that some of the stretches are easier than others, or that you become aware of gentle twinges while you are holding some of the postures. Take all the movements slowly and gently, and never do anything quickly, or anything that hurts. Usually any initial kinks get ironed out as you continue with the stretch routine.

The following two osteopathic stretches are designed to lengthen and mobilise the shorter postural muscles that lie between the individual vertebrae in the spine. Practise them slowly and with care, and feel the wonderful benefits straight away. Use them regularly, and you will be able to chart the changes in your suppleness and ease of movement.

Seated Stretch

Sit with your feet flat on the floor facing forward, and your back straight. You can do this on the side of the bed before getting up in the morning, or later in the day sitting on a chair. Do this very slowly, and you will be able to feel the stretch down almost as far as your toes.

Keeping your back straight, let your chin drop down on to your chest. Place your hands on your head, interlocking your fingers to hold them there securely. Take two deep breaths, and allow the weight of your arms to slowly encourage your head to drop further. Keep your arms relaxed, and as your elbows fall slowly down, take another deep breath. When you notice that your head will sink no further, and your spine is feeling free and relaxed, take another deep breath and as you breathe out, very slowly begin to reverse the process: Lift your elbows out and take the weight back into your arm muscles, and as your head begins to rise, remove your hands and place them at your side.

Let your head continue to come up, and you will notice how light it feels. Let it fall back very slightly — do not lean back and take any tension into your neck — and jut your chin out and up towards your nose. This will gently stretch the muscles at the front of your neck and throat, and down into your upper chest. Hold this position for the length of two deep breaths, then slowly return the head to its normal position.

Standing Stretch

Stand with your back to a wall, with your heels up as close to it as possible, and your feet closer than hip width apart. Keep your arms loosely by your sides. Bend your knees, and pull up on your lower abdominal muscles, so that the natural curve of your low back is flattened against the wall. Allow yourself to travel down the wall until you can go no further without lifting your heels up off the floor.

Let your chin fall gently down on to your chest, and roll your body forwards exquisitely slowly, imagining that you are peeling your spine off the wall one vertebra at a time. Keep your arms loose and relaxed, and let their easy weight help you roll forward. Keep your breathing easy and relaxed, and your movement slow and constant. When you have reached the limit of your stretch, take a deep breath, and just stay there for a moment. Take another deep breath in and, as you breathe out, start to gently stick your vertebrae back to the wall one at a time, slowly and easily reversing your roll, until you are standing up with your spine flat against the wall again and your head up and looking forwards. Gently relax your abdominal muscles, and reintroduce your lumbar curve, and then slowly straighten your legs.

Back Care Rescue Position

If you feel sudden or sharp pain in your back, stop whatever you are doing right away, and get into this Osteopathic Rescue Position as soon as you are able. This is first aid for backs.

Lie on your back on the floor or other solid surface. Bend your knees and bring your heels in as close to your bottom as you can. Then raise your calves up off the floor, supporting them on cushions or pillows, or resting them on the seat of a chair or sofa. Your thighs need to be pointing directly upwards towards the ceiling, and your shins should be lying flat, in the same way as your back is, but higher.

This is a wonderfully comfortable position that will release the lower back and stabilise the whole spine. You can remain in this position for as long as you need to, and can turn your head to watch television, raise your arms to hold a book, etc., so you need not be bored.

If pain persists consult your practitioner.

Massage

Therapeutic massage is a wonderful way to work directly with the muscles and joints and treat them tenderly and effectively. It is a useful way to aid any postural change, and will relieve tired, aching muscles.

A visit to a professional massage therapist is a great gift to yourself. Usually the only people who touch our bodies are parents and lovers, and it is a very healing experience to have someone carefully and expertly work over your body, soothing out any knots, easing out the tensions and generally meeting the skin hunger that we can all experience at times. You can massage yourself whenever you feel tense, or when your muscles have been working hard, or just for the pleasure of it. If you have had a professional massage you will be able to remember some of the techniques that the practitioner used; otherwise the following guidelines will let you begin.

- Always make sure that you are warm — this is especially important because your muscles will tense in the cold.

- Allow enough time. This is a deeply enriching experience, and may be the first time you will have touched yourself lovingly and caringly — make sure you have uninterrupted time in which to enjoy it.
- Never cause yourself pain. This may sound obvious, but if something hurts, you need to stop what you are doing right away. There is never any reason for working through the pain, or persisting to see if it will go away.
- Relax. There is no point in giving your foot a relaxing, caring massage if your shoulders and arms are so tense because you are worried about what you are doing.

You can massage any part of your body that you can easily reach. This means that your whole body with the exception of your back is accessible to your touch. You may want to start simply, choosing an area like your feet, or your face, but it is very easy to develop that into working over a much wider region. Always let your feelings be your guide, and let yourself be carried away.

Choose an oil or a cream to allow your hands to move more freely over your body, as well as for their therapeutic effects. Any moisturising cream can be used, although it will often be quickly absorbed by your skin. Oils will all sit on the skin for a little longer, and allow you to work more easily. Olive oil from your kitchen will do if you have no other — this is a deeply enriching oil that is especially suitable for areas of dry skin, or after exposure to the sun. Other oils you can choose from are available from your chemist or healthfood shop, and include sesame seed oil which is wonderfully warming, and almond oil which is light and beneficial for more tired or sensitive skin.

You can add two drops of essential oil to the oil to gratify your sense of smell and for its therapeutic effects (see page 175). Choose rose essential oil for its deeply feminine qualities and effect on the womb; sandalwood for older skin and to strengthen physical energy; olibanum to ease the emotions, or ylang ylang to stimulate desire.

Make sure that the oil or blend that you are planning to use is warm by placing the container on a radiator, or on top of a hot water bottle. Make yourself comfortable. Keep a towel to hand to mop up any spills, and to cover yourself once you have finished your massage. Begin by tipping a few drops of your oil into your hand, and rubbing your hands together so that they are quite well covered with the oil. Then start to massage your chosen part of the body with slow, easy, gentle rhythmic strokes that move in the direction of the heart. Always move along into the body, towards the heart, even if you are working on your feet. To begin with you will be spreading the oil that is on your hands, and making sure that the area you are massaging is also covered with a light coating of oil. Dip into your container of oil whenever you need to — do not let the area become dry or the strokes will become more difficult, and the effect will be less pleasurable.

Continue stroking lightly, covering every bit of the area you are working on. Imagine getting to know the area with your hands, and following the contours of this body part closely in order to learn as much about it as you can. You can continue stroking and do nothing else, and as you vary the pressure, intensity and speed of each stroke, it will be very beneficial and very enjoyable. Going further, you can choose to use a small, circular movement with your fingers, pressing very lightly into a small area at a time, and then travel on to another spot, pressing very lightly there, and so on. Alternate this smaller, localised stroke with your long sweeping movements. Make sure you use both hands for a sense of continuity and to ensure total coverage of the area — one hand can be supportive while the other is using the circular kneading, then they can both work together in sweeping strokes.

Now begin to use more of your hands, and start to knead gently with the heel of your hand, letting your fingers relax as they rest on top of your body. This is especially nice for large, fleshy areas like big muscles. Keep your movements light. Use both hands to make this more efficient, and for the symmetry it offers. Consider varying the direction in which your hands are moving — perhaps the area you are massaging is large enough to let you work around in a circle, or to take one or more lines along it.

As a rule, the slower your strokes, the deeper you will be able to reach into the muscle and surrounding tissues, and the more relaxing this is likely to be. Long rhythmic strokes, and those that follow the length of a muscle, are most pleasing and relaxing; short, lighter strokes tend to be more stimulating. You may choose to end your massage with some light gentle strokes that just skim the surface of your skin and this will warm and wake up the area. When you are finished, gently hold the area you have been working on for a few moments, then cover yourself up and make sure you stay warm.

Self-massage can form part of your body-care routine, or become one of your regular personal treats. As you become more confident in your skills, you will be able to extend your expertise and include more and more body parts in your massage sessions. You may also like to consider offering a massage to your partner, or to friends.

Working with Energy

There are other ways to work with the energy that is within our body. One of the most enjoyable is through the use of sound. We all express ourselves in this medium every time we open our mouth and speak. Taking this a step further to singing, chanting and toning makes a very personal and effective method of healing. Ancient aboriginal language tells us that to sing is to share our soul. Even those of us who feel we can't sing a note still have our own unique sound to make — a sound that no-one else in the universe can make in the same way. It is our own individual piece of the great harmony that is creation, and we deserve to hear ourselves make that sound.

Simply singing along with a familiar record on the radio can release pent-up emotional energy for us, and those tunes that we tend to sing in the bath or in the shower can be a useful way to balance our energy privately, before we are ready to meet the rest of the world. The ability to make music is really rather special, and it is a shame not to use it. Plants respond to the sounds we make, and I fancy it is rather nice to hum back to bees and sing back to birds on occasion — they give so freely of their own musical talents.

Chanting

Chanting has long been used as a way to focus energy on a particular thing or desire, and one of the simplest chants is the OHM or peace chant:

Stand comfortably, or sit with your spine straight and well supported. Take a deep breath down into the bottom of your belly, and open your mouth wide as though you were gasping in air. Allow the sound of the first syllable to come up from a place deep inside your pelvis, and holding the same breath, become aware of how the sound changes as it travels up your body. Starting with more of an 'ah' sound, it rounds out in the belly to 'aw', becoming an emotional 'ooh' around the heart area. Keep the sound travelling out of your body on your breath, until you reach the end and the 'mmm' sound is coming from near the top of your head. At this point take a large, deep breath and begin again.

Keep the cycle of sound and breath going until you feel you are ready to stop. You will feel quite high — a little light-headed, and usually with a positive feeling ranging from deep contentment to joy and happiness. This is one of the most energising things you can do sitting down, and will astound you in its ability to both energise and relax you at the same time. It is a wonderful thing to do each morning, and forms a lovely part of any meditation or period of quiet reflection.

> Working with the voice is a wonderful aid to anyone with breathing difficulties such as asthma, bronchitis, etc. The discipline of chanting, toning or singing regularly will increase the ability of the lungs, and the ease with which air is expelled from them. These exercises will also aid with the clearing of the sinuses, and can be especially useful if there is congestion, or even after a cold or strong allergic response. I recommend humming to all hay-fever sufferers, and this clears the airways and the sinuses, as well as working out the lungs.
> the ease with which air is expelled from them. These exercises will also aid with the clearing of the sinuses, and can be especially useful if there is congestion, or even after a cold or strong allergic response. I recommend humming to all hay-fever sufferers, and this clears the airways and the sinuses, as well as working out the lungs.

Toning

Toning is a little less structured than chanting. This requires you to allow your body to make whatever sound it feels it needs to. You begin as before by relaxing, and making sure that you are in a comfortable position — lying or sitting are best. This time close your eyes, and become more aware of your own inner reality. Take a breath, and when you are ready, open your mouth and make whatever sound it is that you need to. This might be a sweet, clear note, or something resembling a groan. It can be the sound you need to hear to rebalance yourself, or the sound you need to make and release from your body. You can make a 'la' sound, or use any of the vowel sounds — a, e, i, o, u — or whatever feels appropriate to you.

As before, keep breathing in at the end of each sound that you make, and preparing to make another. Let the connection between your in-breath and your out-breath be flowing and complete, and just let yourself surrender to your own music.

Keep this going for as long as you feel you need to; you will usually find a natural place to finish. Use this as a general exercise to reaffirm your own inner reality and your own power, or make it more specific to how you are feeling by breathing in to a specific place in your body where you are feeling tension, and 'toning' out from that place. You can also use this to work with emotions and memories and release them or bring them to a place of resolution by holding the image in your mind as you tone the energy out of your body.

Dance is another way to work with your body's energy without requiring the use of your vocabulary and critical faculties. Dancing along to your favourite song on the radio is a lovely thing to do, and spending a night out at a dance is terrific exercise for your whole body. Any rhythmic movement can become dance, and you can do it anywhere — to music, or in silence. Nature shows us that there are many different rhythms and movements for our body to make, and this is a wonderfully personal means of expression. Take some time for yourself, in a clear space where you will be able to move freely, and just let yourself go. Your energy might feel young and spring-like, and want to move in large, sweeping gestures; or you may notice a staccato-like beat emerging from part of your body; or the movement may be strange and a little chaotic. Enjoy the luxury of being able to move in whatever way you feel you want to, and make the most of the time and the space that you have. The feelings generated by this type of free-dance are wonderfully healthy and mood-enhancing. I would recommend a daily dose to everyone.

Healing

Healing is, in a sense, what we are all involved with all the time. It is a continuous process within ourselves — the body is engaged in continuous repair and renewal of everything from our hair to our toenails. Healing energy is the energy of life. It exists within and around everyone, and can be used by all of us when we need it. Some individuals are able to tap in to this energy source and work with it for themselves and others; they may call themselves healers. A visit to one of these healers can involve their placing their hands on you, or holding them some distance away from your body. Different healers work in different ways, and healing is not dependent upon time or space, so it works from a distance too.

Healing can occur between lovers, a mother and child, or any individuals who care about each other, and you can witness this for yourself in the loving hug from a caring friend, and the soothing touch of a mother. Essentially it is a matter of energy, and the way in which it can be used. Becoming aware of your own ability to heal yourself is part of your journey through life.

You heal yourself when you choose foods that will promote your health and an environment in which you can be nurtured and grow. Healing yourself energetically means finding a place where you are able to hear, feel, see or perceive what your true needs are, and also perceive how best to meet them.

Discovering this place within yourself is an awe-inspiring journey of self-discovery. You may find it when you meditate, or experience it when you are out in the beauty of nature. Much of our hectic lives can seem to be spent distancing ourselves from our own inner wisdom and source of healing. Modern society can seem unwelcoming to the healer, the Shaman, the wise one and even the individual. The place to begin this epic journey is always with the self. Relaxing and getting to know oneself and one's own real feelings, desires and purpose mark the beginning of the adventure, and the following exercise may be one that you would like to experience for yourself.

HEALING JOURNEYS

You may like to read this through a few times and then embark on the journey by yourself, or you could speak the directions on to a tape, allowing plenty of pauses for you to experience the suggestions, or you may have a friend with whom to do this.

Make some time when you will be able to be quiet and undisturbed. Make sure you are sitting comfortably, and are warm, and have a drink to hand. Close your eyes, take a deep breath in, and as you breathe out, imagine yourself blowing out any tensions and disharmony that you may be feeling. Say to yourself that you are 'safe and secure in your own energy', and mean it. Feel yourself relax as you let your weight become heavy; surrender to the support of the chair behind and underneath you, and to the floor beneath your feet. Take a few deep, easy breaths, and enjoy this experience.

Now use your amazing powers of imagination and your clear ability to visualise to have a wonderful experience. Picture yourself, in your mind's eye, travelling through a familiar landscape that is warm and welcoming. Travel in whatever way you choose, and notice all the small details about the place — the season, the colours, and most importantly how it feels. Enjoy yourself here. Smell the scents that travel on the air, tingle at the gentle touch of your surroundings, and indulge your playfulness. Feel yourself to be there by engaging as many of your senses as you can, and involving your whole body: pick things up with your toes, and feel the breeze in your hair.

A little way ahead is a small clearing, where you will be able to rest for a while and replenish yourself. Notice as you reach this clearing that there is a small dwelling place just inside the entrance. Let yourself relax here, and enjoy the feeling of rejuvenation as you drink in the richness of the atmosphere on every level of your being. After a while you may become aware of a presence — whoever lives in the dwelling may come to visit with you, and if they do they will most surely have a gift to give to you. Take this gift, and say thanks for it. If no-one has appeared, look around the clearing, and see if anything attracts your attention and has been placed there for you. Take this, and give thanks.

Return with your gift, leaving the clearing and travelling back through the familiar landscape until you once again become aware of the floor beneath your feet, and the gentle support of the chair behind and below you. Take some time before you open your eyes, to review your experience and re-examine the gift that you brought back with you.

When you are quite ready, take a deep breath, wriggle your toes and take a sip of your drink. It is a good idea to bring your journey into everyday reality by recording it in some way — perhaps writing the story, drawing or painting some aspects of it, or going and finding some of the items you noticed. Everything that you felt and saw and experienced is important, and all of it from the colours and the scents to the precious gift itself will have layers of meaning for you now and in your future. Capture as much of it as you can to serve as a reminder, and remember too that you may visit that place again whenever you choose to. It is yours.

As you gain confidence in undertaking these inner journeys, and manifesting them in everyday reality, you may choose to explore other regions of your own inner reality. Let your feelings and your own sense of knowing be your guide, and trust to your own ability to always seek out the best for yourself in all that you do.

YOUR OWN MEDICINE CHEST

This is another exercise that is worth experiencing for yoursellf. Take some time to be alone. Sit quietly, and picture or feel any specific aches and pains you may currently have. See yourself as having complete and unhindered access to a magical medicine chest full of elemental healers — light, air, earth, warmth, love, water, movement and a host of other healing salves.

Ask your body what it needs, and allow that energy to heal you. It is as simple as your mind will allow.

Often past conditioning will intervene and the mind will remind you that 'it can't work like that'; 'you are not a healer'; 'healing takes time', or any number of other reasons not to allow full healing to occur. If you can suspend that scepticism for long enough to experience the feelings of this exercise for yourself, you will have begun a profound process of change.

MEDITATION

This is a way of experiencing calm and discovering a still centre within yourself. It can be practised as often or as regularly as you choose, and may form part of your spiritual life, or be used to focus on physical relaxation and mind-body integrity, or as a form of creative problem-solving. Meditation is a strong part of many Eastern spiritual and healthcare traditions, and can take many different forms. The most usual way is while sitting, quite still, with the eyes closed to enable you to focus on your inner world.

To experience this for yourself, make some time when you will be able to relax and will be quite undisturbed. Find a comfortable position in which to sit, making sure that your back is straight and your spine is supported. Close your eyes. You may like to begin by focusing on what you are aware of — the way your body feels, the temperature of the room you are in, any aromas or sounds that you can sense; then develop this following your different senses. Visit your sense of smell, then taste. Notice what you see on the blank screen that your eyelids create for you. Start to become aware of all that you feel, from the fabric of your clothes touching your skin, to the support of the chair or the cushion you are sitting on. Move your awareness so that you can then focus on all the sounds and noises that are around you — from the songs of the birds outside your window to the water moving through the pipes in your house, and the gentle movement sounds that your breath makes as it moves in and out of your body.

You may be surprised at the wealth of information that your body is constantly aware of receiving, monitoring, forming opinions about and assessing — even without any visual input. Spend some time simply recognising this fact, and noticing the busy world of awareness in which you are living. Keep your focus on your breathing and its gentle in and out rhythm.

When you are recording what is going on for your body, your mental processes tend to take second place, but it is worthwhile imagining yourself as a witness in your own mind, and watching the train of thoughts, ideas, images and notions that roll in and out of your conscious awareness.

It can be easy to be seduced by any of these thoughts and ideas, and find that you have spent your quiet, meditative time working on a problem, or exploring a scenario, or reliving an episode that has occurred. The plan, however, was to give yourself time off from this, so endeavour to remain in that witness position, and simply watch the ideas train move on. Remaining focused on your breathing is a good way to do this.

You can feel your connection with the breath that becomes part of you, and moves into and out of your body and your awareness. The air that you breathe in is the same air that surrounds and supports you, touching your skin all over, and reaching out beyond your awareness to fill the rest of the world. Focus on your breath, and allow yourself to really feel it, or become it. Let your mental faculties wonder whether you are air or substance, seated or moving, while you *experience* it. As you become aware of your breath, you can travel with it and reach beyond yourself into the greater world outside, re-experiencing your sense of connection with every living thing. You can also travel deep inside yourself like the air that you breathe in, and experience an end to separation. This is the point at which you are a meditator — the point of bliss, or one-ness; every tradition has its own name for it. This is the point of stillness and peace, where knowing and wisdom are yours.

Meditation occupies a space that is different from ordinary reality, and you may find that you have been sitting for only a few minutes, yet have experienced something that touches infinity. Other times you may sit for a hour or more, and yet still be waiting for the experience. If you are new to this, it is a good idea to make your meditation a regular practice, if possible giving it the same length of time, and the same time-slot each day. Twenty minutes is a good length of time to begin with, and a gentle or music alarm is a lovely way to bring you back into your everyday world.

There are many different ways to meditate. Some schools encourage you to focus on a clear visual image, that will then be retained when you close your eyes, and give you something to anchor yourself in. Others suggest working with the image of a teacher or guru; psychics will often use a candle flame, and Shamans may prefer auditory stimulus. These are all maps, not the territory. It is vital that you find a way that works for you and allows you some 'time off' from everyday, ordinary reality — time to enrich your own inner world, and to bask in the beauty of your own infinite connection with all there is.

Chapter 5

THE ELEMENTS

The elements are present in every aspect of our lives, both in fact and in the symbols they represent for us. In reality, our body is made up of the same elemental factors as the rest of this planet, and its balance, like that of our world, is what constitutes full health. Imagine if the fire from the sun shone a little harder, raising the temperature of the planet by just 10 degrees. Life as we know it would not exist. Similarly in the body, when our inner fire is burning too high and our temperature is raised, we face extinction. If there was 20 per cent more water in this world, our physical form would be considerably different, because we would be living under the sea. When we hold excess water in the body, we completely change the position, constitution and feeling of our inner environment, and the effects can be just as substantial.

Simple headaches will often be cleared by taking a walk in the fresh air. Breathing deeply, and allowing yourself to feel more at home in a natural environment, combine with the rhythmic movements from your walking to ensure a return to harmony for your body. The additional oxygen will clear most headaches. Always choose this cure if your headaches are accompanied by yawning and feelings of stuffiness.

Finding and maintaining a balance between these elements is a part of our healthcare in which we may become consciously involved. A regular contact with the natural world allows us to be reminded of this inner balance, and will go a long way towards ensuring that any insufficiencies are met, quite naturally, and any excesses can be safely expressed. Spending time in nature reminds us of who we are, quite literally. It also heals us in a very direct and simple way — most of us experience this for ourselves quite often when we take an evening walk in order to clear a muggy head, or feel the need to take off for a day in the countryside. Gazing across a natural landscape with its soft lines and gentle edges, colours and shapes does something that is quite unknown in a cityscape. Feeling the touch of the wind on your skin; being able to walk on the soft earth; hearing the sounds of running water and of the animals and creatures that share this planet with us; absorbing the energy of the sun as it reaches deep down inside us to warm and strengthen our bones; sniffing the scent of wild flowers, shrubs and trees as they are carried on the wind like an unexpected gift for the senses; all of these experiences play a part in maintaining our equilibrium and feelings of being alive.

Nature heals us with a touch as soft and gentle as a lover, and does so with a love so unconditional and with which we have such an affinity, that we often do not even recognise it.

Water

Water is a symbol for the strength and generosity of our emotional world. We can use it to represent cleansing, and also as the well-spring of our physical and creative energy. When we gather clutter on an emotional level, it is the same as if it were in a room in our home — things do not run smoothly, and there is an obvious need to clear it. There are many techniques for working with the deeper and occasionally darker emotions, and they certainly are not meant to exist in secret. The simple act of keeping a journal in which you record how you are feeling can do a lot to aid your expression on an emotional level, and keep you in touch with what is going on in your inner world. Often talking out loud about what you feel can be enough to change it and allow you to begin to deal with things more effectively. Whatever means of expression you choose, whether writing, speaking, moving or representing (perhaps through artwork or modelling), the very act of honouring your feelings and emotions is tremendously empowering and can lead to a more open and easy communication within yourself.

This exercise is wonderfully relaxing and can lead to powerful healing responses. You can read this through and remember what to do, or record it on to a tape (making sure to leave plenty of time in between suggestions for you to experience each aspect of the journey), or you may have a friend who would read this for you whilst you relax and enjoy yourself.

Sit comfortably, with your eyes closed, and your body quite relaxed. Imagine yourself in a place in nature, where you feel quite safe and secure. Notice that the sun is gently shining, and you are feeling warm and comfortable. The light is clear enough for you to see by, and you are able to move quite freely. Look over to your right and you will see a small stream of water lazily travelling along the side of the place where you are sitting. In your imagination, get up and walk towards the bank of that stream, and sit down, dangling your feet in the cool sparkling waters. Feel the refreshing coolness of the water, and how it delights your body, and also clears your mind. Feel the water within your body respond to the water in the stream, and feel the affinity that exists between them. Sit there a while and wait to see how your feelings of well-being grow and expand. You may begin to notice other qualities about the water, or see something floating down the stream for you, or appreciate a different aspect of your surroundings. Stay for as long as you feel like luxuriating in the experience.

When you are quite ready, separate yourself from the stream, draw your feet out from the water, and let them dry in the sun. Stay there a while longer enjoying being next to the moving water, and then walk back to the place where you began your journey. Become aware of yourself being back in your room or wherever you are actually doing this, and take a few moments with your eyes still closed to review the events and the feelings that you have experienced. Remember the sensations and how good you felt, and any special points that have meaning for you. When you open your eyes, you may like to record what happened, or share your story with someone. Remember that this is a place to which you can always return, whenever you choose to, and that the feelings and sensations you experienced are a part of you, and can be accessed at any time.

On a practical level, water has an important role to play in our ongoing well-being. We are made up of nearly 80 per cent of water, and we need to ensure an adequate supply of good, clean water every day. Drinking two litres of water each day is a minimum; we need more when the weather is warm, when we exercise, have high protein diets, eat a lot of sweet or salty foods or drink alcohol. Water is essential for a number of different physical functions including food digestion, the elimination of waste from the body, and the circulation of the blood. On a regular day we will breathe out two glasses of water, excrete two glasses through the skin in our perspiration, and route about six glasses through our kidneys. On a hot day, or when exercising heavily, we can use more than three times that amount. (See also Food and Drink, page 85.)

When we are close to a large body of water, we often feel better. This can be a pond, a lake, a stream or river, or the sea. Indoors, this is the bath or the shower; the hosepipe or sprinkler in the summer, and even the running water from the kitchen sink. Spending time close to this element heals that aspect of our lives.

Home Hydrotherapy

Water has many applications: frozen as a first aid measure to relieve pain and help minimise local damage; cold to refresh and cleanse; warm to stimulate and comfort. Ice can be used whenever there is an injury to reduce the risk of bruising and localised swelling, and it also has a numbing effect on the area, thus providing instant pain relief.

> If ice itself is not available, then anything from the freezer will do in its place — frozen peas and corn are especially good because the bag can mould itself easily around the affected limb or joint. Take care when you use a packet of food in this way, because the contents should not be re-frozen, and then eaten. Mark the packet with a clear sign that it is for first-aid use only.

Cold water has traditionally been used to wake up the body and to encourage sluggish circulation. This is especially useful for some people, whose bodies can respond remarkably well to a short, sharp shock. Use cold water as part of your daily bathroom routine to invigorate and refresh any area that you feel is in need. Splashing cold water from the tap onto the face will tighten the skin as well as any toner.

Cold Water Paddling

Cold water paddling is a wonderful wake-up call for the whole body, stimulating general circulation and really drawing your attention all the way down to your feet. This is useful for 'spacer' types, and those whose feet are always cold. Women need to be sure that they do not do it in the week before their period because it is too chilling.

Fill the bath with enough cold water to come up over your ankles, and then walk up and down in it for about 3 minutes. Keep moving, and you will soon feel that the water is not so cold as it seemed in the first shocking moment. When your time is up, sit on the side of the bath for a few minutes, and dry your feet and legs by rubbing vigorously with a towel. You will feel how toasty and warm your feet are, and this is likely to last the whole day. The effects build up if you do this regularly. If you do not have a bathtub, you can use a large washing-up bowl, and walk up and down on the spot.

Another useful way of using the effects of cold water is in contrast with warm. This can be useful for speeding up recovery from injury, and is a gentle but effective way to encourage a fresh supply of blood and nutrients to an area. This will work on every part of your body, from a finger to a limb, and can show equally positive effects when used to treat old injuries or localised arthritic complaints. Simply immerse the affected area in a bowl of warm water, and then move to a bowl of cold water, or use the cold tap. Repeat this as often as you feel able, or have the time for, always finishing with a cold water application. Dry the area well, and repeat as often as possible. If treating a large area — a leg for example — you can incorporate this into your bath-time routine, simply lifting the leg out of the bath when you are at the end of your soak, and spraying with cold water, then putting it back in the bath-water to warm up again, then re-applying the cold water spray. As always, finish with a cold application, and then dry by rubbing vigorously with a towel.

Scottish Douche

The rather strangely named *Scottish douche* is an excellent way to stimulate the nervous system and tone up the whole body. It can be a very useful aid when your system is feeling sluggish, or as part of any detox programme. Used regularly, it can keep your body in good shape, and the effect of the water on your skin and muscles is good for their tone too.

You really need a shower with a detachable head to do this, although similar effects can be obtained with a fixed head shower if you bend your knees and move your body up and down. If you have a friend who can do this for you, so much the better. Run the shower on cold, and taking the shower head in your hand, run it along the length of your spine. Switch to a warmer setting, and feel the contrast as you again run the water down the length of your spine. After 1 minute, turn the water back to cold again. Repeat this as many times as you feel able to, always finishing with the cold spray. Wrap yourself in a towel and sit down for ten minutes after doing this, as the effects can be very stimulating.

Sitz Baths

Sitz Baths work in a similar way, although these are aimed specifically at the pelvic region, and are excellent for waking up and toning the whole area. This makes them a treatment of choice for all sorts of sluggish bowel complaints, and also when there is trouble with painful, irregular or absent periods. Sitz Baths can also be used as part of a treatment regime to encourage the proper functioning of the whole area, and are therefore useful in maximising fertility and coping with any localised dysfunction. Women who feel cold all the time, or whose bottom and hips often feel numb should not do this, but can begin to tone the area using a shower spray that alternates between warm and cooler water. All women need to avoid Sitz Baths in the week prior to menstruation.

You need a bathtub, and a baby-bath or large washing up bowl that is large enough for you to sit in. Fill the bathtub with about twelve inches of cold water. Fill the baby-bath or other container with very warm water, and place it in the bathtub. Sit in the warm baby-bath, with your feet in the bathtub full of cold water. Stay there for about two minutes, then change places so that your feet are in the baby-bath full of warm water, and you are sitting in the bath full of cold water. Stay there for one minute, splashing the cold water to ensure that it covers all your body from the waist down and runs freely in between your legs. Then change places so that you are back in your original position — sitting in the warm water with your feet in the cold. Continue to switch places back and forth as many times as you feel able to, always making sure that you finish with your pelvis in the cold water, and your feet in the warm.

Get up carefully and rub yourself briskly with a towel, especially around your pelvis. Then wrap yourself up well, and sit or lie down for half an hour. You should feel wide awake, with a very clear head, and as though your whole pelvis is warm and toasty. You can do this every other day for three weeks at a time. Take a rest then, and recommence if you want to one week later.

The long term effects can be sensational in terms of improved digestion and elimination, heightened sexual sensitivity and creativity, and general energy levels and feelings of well-being.

Painful periods and symptoms of pre-menstrual syndrome are often relieved when the bowel is clear and the pelvic region is uncongested. Pay close attention to the diet to ensure adequate amounts of plant fibre, and drink plenty of water to stimulate elimination from the bowel. Taking regular Sitz Baths will tone the reproductive organs and can return the area to its own natural cycle. Take Sitz Baths for about one week every month around the time of ovulation to see a positive effect on cramps with the next period. Once the period is due, switch to keeping the whole pelvic area warm, using hot water bottles and sitting in a hot bath whenever necessary.

We must not overlook the positive benefits of simply lying in a warm bath — being able to relax, perhaps in candle-light, and let any cares and tensions float away. Add 2–4 oz of Epsom Salts to ease any aches and pains and improve muscle activity. This is very useful for regulating muscle contraction, and can be helpful if you tend to experience severe cramping or low back pain with a period. Indulge your senses and add two drops to the bath-water of any of the range of pure essential oils — for their aroma as well as their therapeutic effects. (See pages 177–8 for a list of essential oils.)

To relieve the discomfort of cystitis, sit in a bath of warm water to which you have added a handful of sea salt. Make sure that you drink as much water as you can manage, and remain in the bath to pee (it will make it less painful). Ensure that the level of the bath water comes up over your kidneys, and keep the temperature high enough to be comfortable. Sip some unsweetened Cranberry juice to flush out your system, and make sure you follow good hygiene measures scrupulously to prevent further infection. This means always wiping from front to back when you go to the toilet, not using internal sanitary protection or any perfumed products around the genitals, and showering before sex and peeing as soon as decently possible afterwards.

Water is a wonderful medium for carrying remedies into our body. The old fashioned *steam inhalation* is a wonderful way to cleanse the skin on the face and neck, and can prove a fast and effective remedy for colds, stuffy headaches, sinus congestion and sore throats.

Fill a large bowl with boiling water, and place it on the table. Sit in front of it, covering the bowl with a towel, and placing another one around your neck. Take a deep breath, then lift the towel from the bowl and place your head inside this steamy tent. Keep your breathing slow and shallow at first, and come up for air if it starts to feel too hot or claustrophobic. Stay in the 'tent' for as long as you are able, or until the steam no longer rises from the surface of the water.

Add some sage leaves to the water to relieve a sore throat, eucalyptus leaves or a sprig of fresh rosemary to clear the sinuses, and a few slices of lemon and a clove to get rid of a cold.

Fire

This element has come to symbolise so much for us, ranging from the myth of Prometheus to the passionate and often mercurial nature of our sexual desire. In our modern lives we do not often come into contact with fire — it is no longer at the centre of our homes keeping us warm and providing the fuel for us to cook with. Fire in our lives is often hidden behind radiator grills, stored in underground boilers or blown at us through heating systems. We rarely have an opportunity to glimpse the flames and follow the dance they make as they flash and burn and weave, crackling as they transform matter into something invisible. Sitting in front of an open fire is a wonderfully magical and soothing thing to do. The blaze emits a huge number of negative ions that will relax and calm the physical senses, while the magnetism of the fire itself settles the mind. Seers and psychics often work with flames for divination and problem solving, and you can sample this for yourself the next time you are close to a fire. Just relax and allow your mind to work with the flames to bring whatever is needed to your conscious awareness. Notice what you see and allow the changing shapes and forms that appear in and around the fire to inform and inspire you.

One way to bring fire safely indoors is with candles. These can be used to experience the type of seeing-exercise mentioned above, and provide a very good focus for any type of meditation or psychic focusing. Sit in front of a lit candle and allow yourself to stare through the flame, letting your eyes and your attention be touched by the light, but travel on through it. Just sit and look, and keep your mind open so that you can recognise and process whatever you see or sense. Give yourself as much time as you need, and relax into reaching through the fire, letting yourself go and experiencing a whole new sense. Once you are used to working with the candle flame in this way, try the following exercise to refine your technique: Look around the flame — shift the focus of your eyes so that you can see the whole of the outline of the flame, without seeing *it*. Once you begin to do this you will usually become aware of a colour or colours surrounding the flame that are not always visible through normal or everyday sight. Work with these colours by allowing them to expand and change, and see if you can move them through all the colours of the rainbow and then back again to the colour that fire first showed to you.

Candles will throw a wonderfully restful light on any activity, and can be a marvellous addition to the relaxation effects of a soak in a warm bath. They will tend to change the atmosphere of a room, too, making it soothing or romantic. They are a wonderful way to augment the wind-down process at the end of the day, and can add the missing element to relaxation before going to bed. Always keep a candle by your bedside, to light before preparing for bed, and also to use for its gentler glow in place of electricity should you wake in the night.

Another way to bring fire into the home is to let the air carry it — simply opening the doors and windows on a sunny day will bring sunshine into the room. This can change even the dullest corner into a wonderful energy-giving source of light and colour. Spending time in the sunlight is profoundly important for the body. The skin will react and experience changes, Vitamin D is produced, and there is a general feeling of well-being. The strong effects of sunlight, as it touches the eyes and seems to reach deep down into our bones, can be an immediate counter-effect to a long winter and to feeling emotionally low, or experiencing low energy levels. It is important to stress here that it takes very little exposure to sunlight in order to experience these benefits. Proper care and protection need to be employed whenever we expose our vulnerable selves to the full force of the sun's energy. Never spend time outdoors when the sun is at its strongest without full cover and/or protection — rather enjoy the light and the warmth at more suitable times of day.

Whenever there is an atmosphere of energy, enthusiasm, excitement and movement, then elemental fire is present. This can be channelled into all aspects of life from personal and creative endeavours to a more general approach to work and relationships. Fire is the wonderful sense of adventure that we can discover in even the most mundane activities, and it is the excitement we feel when we greet a friend. It can move us to be expansive and generous in our physical lives and in all our dealings, and to reconnect with the joy that is in our hearts. It is always ready to dance its way into the rest of our lives.

The following exercise will enhance your feeling of being in touch with your own sexual and creative energy.

Belly Dance

Stand with your feet flat on the floor, about shoulder width apart, and your knees very slightly bent, or 'soft'. Begin to move your pelvis in a figure eight movement, and increase the movement until it is as fluid and expansive as feels comfortable. Close your eyes and become aware of this flowing movement as you move your hips, outlining the symbol of infinity. Make a figure eight movement with your hands and arms, and let the energy that is settled in your pelvis spread throughout your body, moving your shoulders, your head, your eyes, every part of you with its silky, sensual energy. Keep moving in this way, becoming the movement and allowing it to flow through and around you as you describe your energy through the space you are in.

If you have a favourite piece of music, you might like to play it while you do your figure eight dance.

Dance for as long as you feel moved to, and repeat this every day to enhance its effects.

Fire is the energy of light and colour therapy. These are finding an enormous number of health applications, ranging from their ability to improve skin complaints to their effectiveness against forms of depression and Seasonally Affected Disorder. You can experience this for yourself by discovering what colour or colours your body responds best to. This may well change according to your feelings, the seasons, your energy levels and where you are in your menstrual cycle. Bring this energy into your life in the simplest of ways by allowing yourself to be drawn to a particular colour, or spectrum, and make the basic colours welcome in your wardrobe and in your home. Include a place that is blue, where you can feel the stillness and calmness of water; a yellow area for you to be warmed and inspired; red accents to remind yourself of the spark of life; a green space where you can experience renewal; mauves and pinks to enhance your feelings of love and your ability to communicate, and whatever other colours you can identify or want to have around you. You do not have to change the decorations in order to honour all these colours. Group a few objects together in one place to give a strong effect and add flowers, a plant or a picture to enhance it.

Experience your own inner fire through the following exercise:

Energetic Fire

Sit comfortably and close your eyes. Picture yourself on a warm sunny day, sitting outside under a gorgeous blue sky, with a few floating clouds. Hear the distant sounds of children at play, and feel the sense of adventure that is in the air. Take a deep breath in, and feel how wonderful it is to be alive. Bring to mind a time when you felt happy and relaxed and easy like this, and were able to share that happiness with a friend. Re-experience the joy that you felt in sharing and expressing your happiness as you re-run that time in your mind's eye. Open your eyes and let the feeling stay with you.

The physical fire in your body can be experienced whenever you feel energy rise up and move you forwards — this can be when you use your creative or sexual energy or when you feel inspired or enthused about anything. Fire is a great transformer of energy, and is often used to represent the digestive system and its clear ability to alter the raw materials with which we fuel the body into the energy that we need for all our endeavours. This mysterious alchemical process occurs within us every day, without our even needing to recognise it. We can honour this process by making sure that we eat regularly, so that the flames have something to consume, and that we allow the fire to burn well without dousing it or adding anything that will make it burn too strongly.

The digestive fire within the body reaches a peak around noon, along with that other representative of fire that is present in all our lives, the sun. Flooding a flame with cold water will put it out, and this is exactly the effect on our digestive ability if we start a meal with an iced drink or anything too cold. Pouring alcohol on a fire will make it flash and burn too quickly — possibly burning itself out if it does not have enough solid fuel to sustain it. Apply this message to your own habits, and consider the effects of alcohol on your digestion, especially in relation to mealtimes. Consider too the effects of food on this element — does your body need the fiery heat of a chilli or the supportive warmth of some fresh ginger root? Or would your digestive system respond best to the cooling effects of some ground coriander seeds, or a cup of mint tea?

Ask yourself how fire manifests itself in your body, and in your life. Do you feel cold, or is there any evidence of hot, red skin rashes; have you the enthusiasm and energy you need to feel inspired about something; can you enjoy yourself and share this energy with others; are you able to express yourself creatively and sexually? Sexual and creative expression are perhaps the most 'fiery' of our inner drives, and certainly those that can be fast moving in their appearance, and warming and deeply satisfying when they are in balance. Allow time for these energies to manifest themselves in your life, and you will experience the joy that comes from keeping a well-stoked fire at the centre of your physical home.

Air

Air is all around us all the time, touching every part of us at any one time — gently embracing our skin, and filling our body with each breath. Air can also represent the power of the mind, and this has a wonderful role to play in our own healthcare. The way we think impacts directly on the way we feel, and vice versa. Our mind is one of our strongest and most faithful allies when we work with it to improve our health and well-being. You will know for yourself how fantastic a response you can get when you concentrate fully, and focus on achieving a particular outcome. Imagine turning this incredible ability onto your quest for full health and happiness, and you can expect to experience all that you think you can. Literally. Whatever we can envisage for ourselves is possible for us to experience for ourselves. Obviously, you can carry an image of Arnold Schwarzeneger in your mind for ever, and if your genes say you look like Groucho Marx, then that's who you look like. Beyond the impossible, though, an amazing array of options exists, and all we need to do is to tap into our reserves and be prepared to experience the change.

When you picture something happening to yourself in your mind's eye, your body responds in much the same way as if it was happening in reality. Therefore, you can achieve the changes that you need to make by bringing your mind on board as co-worker in every project you undertake. Research shows that you get better results when you involve your mind, and this can be seen in everything from weight-training (where you picture the increase in muscle size as you are performing the exercises) to sex.

An everyday way to use this wonderful facility is to be aware of our attitude towards every aspect of our life, from the way we do things to the way we speak and move our body. Stop and think for a moment about the things you say about yourself — do you talk disparagingly about parts of your body? And what about your expectations for your life? Do you assume that bad luck will occur, or expect to fail, or experience pain in your dealings with the world or with others? Imagine turning that right around: becoming your own thought police and ensuring that all your thoughts, ideas and notions were as affirming, positive, supportive and life-enhancing as they could possibly be. Try this for yourself, first simply listening or witnessing your own inner voice and registering how positive or negative it is, and then turning any pessimistic, sceptical or invalidating trains of thought into strong endorsements of who you are and how you choose to be.

Structure this positive thinking by using affirmations, or positive thought repetitions. These are like special ideas that you can plant inside your head, and repeat to yourself as often as you remember. They can be about anything at all that you wish to change or improve in yourself and your world. The most all-inclusive one is 'Every day in every way I am getting better and better', but you can make one that is totally specific and special to you, and that will work more successfully for you because it is personal. Think this thought of affirmation whenever you have a spare moment, and write it down so that you can read it and see it too. Treat it like the lines you may have received as a punishment in school — repeating it over and over again, so that you will *really* get the message.

You can use these affirmations to work for change in any area of your life, from specific physical concerns to the way you react to stressful situations, or your mind-set on any issue. Find ways to enjoy this mental work-out, and to make it as rewarding as possible: make your affirmations fun and silly, or include rhyme in order to imprint it on your subconscious more easily. Set your affirmations to music if that is what moves you, or flesh out all the details in glorious living colour. Use whatever skills you have to develop in whatever way you feel you need to.

One of the mind's great abilities is that of being able to visualise things so strongly that the body can believe they are real. This faculty is the route to our being able to have a great time, without going anywhere or taking anything, and also makes it possible for us to alter the way we feel both physically and emotionally. Visualising something is a wonderful aid to the words of any affirmation. It is also a powerful technique that can be used on its own for relaxation, pleasure and continued good health. Imagine going inside your body and seeing yourself meeting and greeting your immune system, being able to picture it in whatever form you see it functioning. Now when you face the flu season, or feel a cold coming on, you *know* exactly what you need to make happen internally to keep yourself well. You can use this facility to enjoy your relaxation too, by picturing yourself in a quiet, restful setting where you are experiencing something beautiful and self-enhancing. The more you work at this, the better you get, and the more impressive the results. Making your mental work as rich and resonant as possible will improve your move towards an optimum outcome, so include all the detail that you can, involve your senses, your memory, tactile skills, and everything else that you can.

On a physical level, our greatest contact with the element of air is through the breath. The way we breathe is not something we often think about. Stop for a moment right now and notice how fluid your breathing pattern is, and how deeply you take each new breath of fresh air into your body. When we are tense, or concentrating, or simply through habit pattern, our breathing can become shallow and erratic.

Easy Relaxed Breathing

Easy relaxed breathing is important to every aspect of our lives. Taking full, deep breaths will relax you and serve as a natural break from whatever you are doing. It will open your ribcage, release tension in your neck and shoulders, and give you a gentle, internal massage. This is also great exercise for your abdominal muscles. Breathe this way for five minutes every day, and it will soon become your natural breathing habit.

Sit down in a comfortable chair with your feet flat on the floor and your back straight and well supported. Place your left hand on your belly, and your right hand on your upper chest, just below your neck. Relax. Take a few breaths, and notice your normal breathing pattern. Most people's right hand will be moving up and down, and their left hand will be quite stationary.

Now picture yourself taking each full, new breath deep down into your abdomen, and breathe right out from there too. Feel your whole body respond to your new gentle breathing rhythm, and experience the relaxation and renewed energy that come from that. See your midriff and abdomen expand as you take in each new, full breath, and flatten as you breathe out. Your left hand will be moving in and out with each breath, and your right hand will stay quite still.

Circular Breathing

Circular breathing is a wonderful exercise for bringing calm to the whole system. It can be done as a prelude to any form of relaxation or gentle exercise, or to calm and steady oneself, or as part of a meditation. It is especially useful as a way to centre one's energy and remember the strength and security that comes from being a part of a natural cycle. The physical benefits are legion, and this is a tremendously beneficial exercise for anyone with breathing difficulties, a history of chest congestion or a desire to open up their emotions. I could wax on about the myriad advantages of this exercise, and it really is one of my all-time favourites; I am quite sure it will benefit just about everybody, and assist with almost all concerns.

Begin by making sure you are in a comfortable position, either sitting or lying down with your back straight. Place the palm of your left hand over a spot in the middle of your abdomen, just below your belly button. This is the physical centre of gravity in your body, and is traditionally regarded as a reservoir of energy for the whole system. In Eastern traditions it is known as Hara, or Tan Chien. Cover your left hand with your right. This will now serve as a focus for your breathing, and as a filter — you are going to see yourself breathing directly into this place. Many breathing exercises extend the depth of the breath, and some encourage holding the breath too, but this is the only one I know of that honours all points in the breathing cycle, and makes space for you to stay empty.

The cycle has four stages, and you can count to four at each stage to keep yourself in rhythm, and to balance each quarter of the circle. Start by breathing in to the count of four, then hold your breath for a count of four, breathe out for a count of four, and stay empty for a count of four. Then breathe in to a count of four, and keep the circle going, following the same routine until you feel yourself reach a natural close. See yourself breathing right in to that place just below your belly button, and enjoy the feelings of exploring the full range of your breath, and the feelings and sensations that you are experiencing. Do not strain or hold any tension, simply allow the count of four and the four directions to guide your breath.

Air Baths

Air baths are another way to enjoy the touch of air within and around us. Take off all of your clothes and stand close to an open window in the warm weather, or near an open inside door during the cooler months — anywhere you can feel a light breeze of air. Stand there for a moment and enjoy the feeling of letting your skin breathe, and having the gentle breeze touch you all over. Your skin will love this. Then imagine you are having a shower in this fresh, clean air, and use your hands to 'splash' it all over and around your body. Take an air bath every day to waken up your skin and improve your sense of your body and general physical ease.

> Working to improve the breathing ability of the skin takes the pressure off the other main breathing organ, the lungs. All these measures to improve skin function will open up a new avenue of elimination for your body. They are especially useful if there is a history of bronchitis, asthma, or breathing difficulties brought on by allergies, airborne pollutants and anxiety attacks.

Skin Brushing

Skin brushing directly wakes up your body all over. It is a wonderful skin softener, and stimulates the circulation as well as giving the lymphatic system a real boost. If you skin brush regularly, you will notice a marked change in your pattern of perspiration — it will be lessened, and the odour will change to become much less strong. You will also need to use less soap on your body, because the brushing has the effect of cleansing your skin and opening all your pores, to ensure freer elimination. You can do this every day — make it part of your bathroom routine, and combine it with cold water paddling (see page 130) or another hydrotherapy technique to maximise the positive effects.

To do this you will need a natural bristle brush with a removable handle. Stand naked, and begin brushing on the soles of your feet. You will soon find out what degree of pressure feels best, but you will be surprised at how briskly you can brush, and how much your skin will like it. Brush up your legs and all the way up your body — over your hips and around your bottom, up over your abdomen towards your heart. Brush up your trunk and then over both your hands, up both arms and across your shoulders, always brushing towards your heart. Then put the handle in and brush up your back. When you have finished you can brush over your scalp, and down your neck. Avoid the skin on your face which is a little too sensitive. You will feel energised, clear-headed and very refreshed.

Make sure you spend some time each day giving yourself the freedom to experience breathing as good a quality of air as you can manage. This may mean taking a walk in a park or a wood, or even along a tree-lined avenue, and making sure that you escape as far as possible from any traffic fumes and other airborne pollutants. Each breath you take oxygenates your blood, ensuring that your body receives the best possible nutrient mix in order to work at its best, perform well, and repair itself efficiently; it supplies your brain with the raw ingredients it needs in order to think and reason to its optimum. When every breath is as clean and pure as you can possibly make it, then you give yourself one of the best possible chances for full health.

Earth

The element of earth is represented all around us in the soil. It is the medium for growth, and this is also represented as how we see the body. A regular contact with the earth is important for full health, and this can be achieved by simply spending time out of doors, walking on the earth, or by more actively communing with it through outdoor pursuits like gardening.

The earth can represent our ability to transform things, and is our physical home, akin to the way that the body is the physical home to our spirit. Whenever we nurture and nourish ourselves and our environment we are communing with earth symbolically. Earth is a wonderful transformer of energy, again in the same way as the body is — changing simple ingredients like foods into energy for movement and growth.

Ground yourself to increase your sense of being in your body, and your ability to be physically responsive. This is a good way to stop any 'spaceyness' or a tendency to be stuck in your head. The following exercises all serve to remind you of your physical home, and how great it can feel to be fully present within it:

- Stand with your feet flat on the ground and about shoulder width apart. Close your eyes and feel how free your spine is, reaching right up through you and down to your base. Imagine that you have a tail that is just a continuation of your spine, and that carries on down from it, reaching down to the floor, down into the ground, down through the upper layers of the earth, and down right to the centre of this planet. When there, it discovers its own hook to wrap around and hold it fast. See how your energy feels now that you are firmly anchored to the centre of the earth.
- Stand with your feet flat on the floor, quite wide apart. Lift your arms so that they extend out on either side of your head, and your body forms an 'X' shape. Close your eyes and become aware of the earth energy that is below your feet. Allow it to reach up through your body, starting at the soles of your feet and travelling all the way up to your belly button. Hold it there for a moment to really feel its effects in your body, then allow it to continue up your body and up your arms till it is in your hands, and extending out beyond you to touch the energy above you. Now become aware of the energy of the heavens that is above your head. Allow it to fall softly into your body, starting with your hands and travelling all the way down to your heart. Hold it there for a moment to really appreciate its wonder, then allow it to continue down your body and into your legs, until it reaches your feet and extends down beyond you to contact the earth. Become aware of your role as conduit for heavenly and earthly energy, and allow them to mix within you, as you

walk on the earth with your body and touch the heavens with your head.

The earth comprises a range of coverings, from the rich lush grasses that cushion our steps to the sand crystals that exercise every muscle in our feet. Walk on as many of the earth's surfaces as you can to enrich your experience, and as a work-out for your body.

Stones and crystals carry the energy of the earth, and can help us balance and remember ourselves. They can be worked with in a number of ways to heal different aspects of ourselves, and people often feel better when they are around. Different stones and crystals will have different effects on us, and it is important to give yourself time to choose a stone to act as your companion or healer at any time. Some people would say you should give yourself time to allow the stone to choose you.

- Rose quartz has an affinity with the heart and the emotions, and is useful for balancing feelings and enhancing love and generosity.
- Jade is an effective healer for the pelvis and will regulate sexual energy and enhance creativity.
- Diamonds have a connection with the third eye and can help clear any lack of connection with our own inner knowing.
- Amethyst can clear the mind and aid clarity of thought.

> If you experience shock, or any sudden event that startles you and leaves you feeling unsettled, look around to see whether there is any stone nearby. Take the stone, and hold it in your hands immediately over the point just below your belly button which is the centre of all your physical energy. Hold it there while you breathe deeply; allow the energy from the stone to bring you back safely into yourself and remind your body energy of the richness of being grounded and alive. Breathe with the stone for as long as you feel you need to, and then return it to the place where it was sitting.

Salts are also representative of the earth, and can be used to carry all the cleansing and transformational energy of the earth, enabling it to be used more easily.

Add a handful of salt to a basin of water and soak your feet in it. Allow the salt to draw any impurities and negative energy out from your body and transform them into neutral energy in the solution of the water. Do this at the end of the day when you are feeling hassled and weary, and witness the transformational powers of the earth for yourself, as you feel your body being cleansed.

Feeling at home here in this physical incarnation is a powerful way to honour the element of earth. Deal with it practically by taking to the earth anything that you are having trouble with, and allow it to transform it for you.

Find a piece of ground where you will be safe and undisturbed. This might be in your garden or in the countryside. You might like to ask a friend to keep watch over your space if you are in public to make sure that you will be able to complete this exercise without being troubled in any way. Ask them to sit out of easy listening distance, so that you will be free to experience all that you need to without concern that you may be overheard.

Begin by looking around you and noticing all that you see, then lie down on the ground, pressing your belly to the earth and renewing the connection between you and the earth at this key spot. Your umbilicus is the point where you were once joined to your mother and through which you received all the nourishment you needed. Lying in this way allows you to recognise the earth as your mother, and to feel the deep tie that exists between you.

Relax, enjoy the feelings of becoming reacquainted with the earth in this way, and then dig a small hole near your head. You are going to tell the earth about something that is troubling you, or that you are having difficulty dealing with, or simply need to share. Speak your story into the hole, knowing that you are talking directly into the ear of the earth, and that she is listening. Talk for as long as you need to, and fill in all the details so that your story is as complete as it needs to be. Tell the earth how it feels, what your concerns and desires are, and how best you feel you can be assisted. Talk about anybody else who is involved, and speak as freely as you possibly can — the earth will keep your secret. When you have finished your story, wait for a moment or two and see whether there are any additional facts or details that you have omitted. When you are certain that your story is complete, cover in the hole and sit up. Look around you and see whether there is anything that catches your eye —

a stone, a leaf, or a flower perhaps. Give yourself time to see if anything appears different since you arrived at that place.

If it feels appropriate to do so, pick up the item that caught your attention and take it with you when you leave. If nothing special called to you, then simply thank the earth for listening, and leave the place as you found it. It is a good idea to forget that site, or at least the spot where you dug your listening hole. Over the next few weeks, be watchful and be prepared to witness the changes that can occur within this area of your life that you have shared with the earth. If you carried something away with you from your time communing with the earth, keep that as a focus for whatever new things may come into your life as a result of your having let go of your story.

Balancing the Elements

Many traditions work with a circle or wheel as a means of portraying the way the elements contribute to our lives. This a good symbol from which we can see ourselves as being in the centre of the wheel or circle, and the various elements as having positions around its rim. When we are in the centre of our circle, we can turn to see any point on its edge, and have the ability to move in any direction. If an area or element is out of balance, it will alter the way the whole wheel turns, and only when we are at centre can we determine our own sense of balance and what we need to move forward.

Consider drawing the wheel of your own life right now, and placing the elements within it. Do this physically, either drawing or painting a circle on paper, or constructing it with any variety of things that will represent your reality. Work with this in any way that comes most easily to you — making lists around the circle, using signs and symbols, or placing articles in whatever place is most meaningful. You are constructing a medicine wheel, and the medicine you will receive is through your view of what your life is like right now. Do this indoors or out of doors, wherever you feel most comfortable, and allow it to be as special, enlightening and transformational an experience as you need it to be.

Ask yourself where you would be sitting — at the centre or somewhere on the periphery. Include as many aspects and facets of your life as possible, including where you wish to be, as well as where you are, and where you have come from. If earth sits at one point on your circle, and opposite it is fire, know that when you are sitting within earth, it is the illumination of fire that inspires you and fills your vision of the future. When you are sitting in the element of water, see that it is the knowledge and wisdom of air that is ahead of you. Whenever you travel to the limit of your experience in any one direction, and turn and sit there to become comfortable, then you are already facing in the direction of your return. This is part of the paradox of taking responsibility for your life, and can also yield tremendous comfort.

When your physical and emotional health is at a point that you can recognise as being settled in any one direction or element, the symbol of your life as a wheel or circle can remind you that the answer to what you need is likely to be right in front of you. Living at the centre of the wheel of your life means being able to command all the energy at your disposal, and being able to respond.

If you feel that you are not in control, consider the weight of each element in your life to date, and in your world right now. Perhaps you could change your focus, or shift the weight of your activities to achieve a greater balance and bring yourself back to the centre. If you are being over-emotional, consider the fluid, flowing qualities of water that can help you travel on and into a new place. When you feel stuck physically, remember the transformational powers of the earth, and enlist her help to change where you are right now. Get to know your own favoured elements, or those with which you feel most at home, and seek to develop any other directions that will round out your experience, and enable your journey through life to be less wobbly.

Chi Dynamics Exercises

These are a wonderful system of healthcare measures, exercises and postures that derive from Eastern traditions, and have been formulated into a plan for ongoing health. Perform the following exercises every morning, or whenever you feel the need to connect with a particular element, or balance it.

Warming Up

Stand with your feet together and bend your knees. Place your hands on your thighs, about two thirds of the way down, and rest them there. Look forward at a point on the floor about six feet in front of you, and keep your neck relaxed. Circle your knees around to the left, keeping them together, and your feet flat on the floor. Repeat this eight times, then circle them around to your right eight times.

Straighten up, and move your feet to about hip width apart. Bend your knees so that you drop down by about 2 inches. Keep your feet facing forward or slightly turned out, and flat on the floor. Raise your hands up so they are in front of your heart, with your elbows raised also, and push them slowly out in front of you while you breathe out, then part your hands and let them travel around and back to your heart while you breathe in. This is just like a breast stroke movement in swimming. Repeat eight times.

WATER

Do your warm-up exercises, then stand with your feet about hip width apart and facing forwards or slightly outwards. Hold your hands loosely on your abdomen, just below your belly-button. Turn your body to the left and reach out with your hands to describe a small pool of water just by your side. Bend down to it, and imagine gathering up two handfuls of the water and draw them up your body to 'rinse' your face. Allow your body to bend backwards slightly as you reach your head. Make this movement while you are breathing in. Then sweep the water off your body back down to the pool, straightening up as you do so, and bending down again as the water falls off. Breathe out through your mouth while you do this, and the sound you make will be rather like a 'Chee'. Repeat this three times, then turn your body to the right, and cleanse this half of you in exactly the same way.

Fire

Do your warm-up exercises, then stand with your feet about hip width apart, and facing forwards or slightly outwards. Turn to your left side, and imagine that you are looking into the sun. Raise both your arms towards it as you breathe in. Your left arm will be reaching out beyond your body, and your right arm will lie across your body. Imagine you are gathering some of the energy of the sun, and drawing it down through your body to the earth as you pull your left arm down, drawing your elbow in to your waist, and follow the same line with your right arm so that it is pointing down towards the ground. Breathe out through your mouth as you do this. Repeat the exercise three times, then turn to the other side and draw the fire through you from that direction in exactly the same way.

Air

Do your warm-up exercises, then stand with your feet about hip width apart, and facing forwards or slightly outwards. Hold your hands loosely just below your belly-button, and bring them circling out around the side of you to meet in the midline again just above your head while you breathe in. Hold them there for a brief moment, before drawing them both back down the centre of your body to that point below your belly-button. Breathe out through your mouth as you draw your hands down, and hold them there for an instant to enable the energy from the air around you to collect and settle. Repeat this exercise as many times as you feel moved to.

EARTH

Do your warm-up exercises, then stand with your feet about hip-width apart, and facing forwards or slightly outwards. Hold your hands loosely just below your belly-button, and lean forwards slightly as you let them describe a circle around you, reaching back to your low-back. Draw your arms up your body from your kidney area, up to your armpits, and then straighten your arms up into the air above your head and slightly out to your side. Make this complete movement while you are breathing in, then draw your arms together and down the centre of your body to that point below your belly-button. Breathe out through your mouth as you draw your hands down, and hold them there for an instant to enable the energy you have gathered up from the earth and drawn through your body to collect and settle. Repeat this exercise three times.

When you have finished the exercises, stand still for at least a minute to feel your energy settle and stabilise before moving off. Keep your hands gently held in the midline, symbolising the way your body stores this energy at that point.

Chapter 6

NATURE'S GIFTS

However good your overall health, there are times when a little extra support is needed. There are also occasions when your body could use a bit of a fillip, or some additional help to get over a particular stage of an illness, or an extra push towards greater health and well-being. Nature makes available to us a wide range of potential remedies and cures. Beyond the natural good sense measures of Nature Cure that can be found in the rest of this book, the following cures are for use whenever there is an additional need. They are the gifts of nature. They have truly beneficial side-effects, such as their balancing effect on the system. The powerful sense that we are treating ourselves quite naturally, and taking responsibility for our own healthcare, is a strong healer.

- **Herbs** are the natural extension of the fruits and vegetables that we eat in our everyday diets. Including them in meals and drinks for their specific healing values makes them an absolute medicine. They can also be of assistance when made into a tisane, a compress, gargle, poultice or inhalant (see the Kitchen Pharmacy, page 194.) Herbal remedies work very well with the physical body.

- **Flowers** and the remedies that can be made with them impart both their nutritional values and their energy in order to work well as emotional balancers. These can be used in a number of ways according to need, from bringing beauty into our lives to taking drops of the remedy on the tongue.
- **Essential oils** remind us of the pleasure of enjoying a treatment; they stimulate our senses as well as lending their therapeutic value. Their myriad applications make then an especially versatile remedy. They work on both physical and emotional levels.
- **Tissue salts** are often used to supplement the diet and are a strong support throughout the range of health concerns that we all face. They can often address specific nutritional imbalances as well as dealing with a range of symptoms.
- **Nutritional supplements** serve to support our best dietary intentions, and fill the gap between what we eat and optimum nutrition. They serve to strengthen the physical body.

Treat all these remedies as medicines, being respectful and mindful of their strength and efficacy. The worst thing that you can do is to treat them as harmless, and to take them carelessly. Their greatest strength is that they work so effectively with the subtler systems of the body, and this is an area where results are profound, if sometimes slower to manifest. Follow the directions for use in each section, and always trust your own intuition. The recommended dosages are extremely conservative, and will be suitable for psychics and other sensitives. Whenever you take a remedy, monitor your reactions. Stop taking it if you experience any negative reaction, and seek the support of your natural healthcare practitioner.

Herbs

Herbs can be used in a variety of ways to augment our overall health, and as specific remedies for particular symptoms or complaints. Adding them to the diet is one of the simplest and most effective ways to benefit from their health-giving properties. They can also be taken as simple teas or infusions, and in cordials, and used externally as poultices and compresses, creams and ointments, or applied directly to the skin.

> Crush a fresh angelica leaf and place in the front of the car when travelling on long journeys to prevent travel sickness. This is especially good for children, but works for all the car's occupants.

Herbs form the basis of many of the pharmaceutical drugs that we use as modern medicines, and they are still being explored to develop cures for a wider range of illnesses and complaints. The nicest thing about taking herbs in their natural form is that they are made available to us as nature intended: in a complex mix with other active ingredients that will balance and improve the effects of the individual remedy. They are safe to take in this way because the active ingredient is usually present only in amounts that the body can use or respond to, unlike the isolated, refined and synthesised version that is delivered in drugs.

> Place a teaspoon of dill seed in a cup of hot water, and leave to stand for five minutes. Strain the liquid and cool. Add a little honey or sugar to taste, and you have gripe water, without the alcohol. This will settle and soothe a range of stomach and digestive complaints, and is a wonderful treatment for infants.

Herbs can safely and effectively be combined with other healthcare measures, including vitamin therapy and the use of remedies such as essential oils. It is generally advisable to take herbs individually if you are treating yourself at home, although if you are adding the plants to your meals, trust your digestion to filter out any excess, and add as many as you feel drawn towards.

To take as a remedy, consider eating the fresh herb, and if that is not possible due to the season, or desirable (some taste too bitter or unpleasant), then the dried herb is the next best choice. This can be sprinkled on to food near the end of the cooking time, or made into a tisane or infusion by covering with just-boiled water and leaving to steep for a few moments before drinking. When neither the fresh nor dried herb is available, consider taking the tincture. This is the essence of the herb which has been extracted and distilled, and preserved in alcohol. I do not recommend this method for everyone because of the alcohol, nor do I suggest its long-term use. Tinctures make an effective way of storing herbs, and are suitable for all external applications. Herbs are also available in tablet form, and this is a convenient way to take them, but be certain that they are tableted with only natural ingredients. You do not want to take a tablet that includes sugar, flavourings, colourings, dyes and preservatives; you just want the herb.

> Saw Palmetto berries are a wonderful remedy for prostate enlargement. This affects 80 per cent of men over 45, and causes a range of problems from low sperm production and infertility to difficulty peeing. Take 300–600 mg of Saw Palmetto berry in tablet form each day, and work with the diet, hydrotherapy and exercise to improve the tone of the area. Include pumpkin seeds and oily fish in the diet, and avoid pesticides and wheat bran.

Herbs make an excellent first-aid treatment for all the family. Children can safely be treated with fresh herbs, and with dried herbs that are made into teas; reduce the strength accordingly. They will also respond very well to external applications, so use a weak tea to wash the skin, or add to bath-water. Do not give herbal tablets or tinctures to children without the advice of your natural healthcare practitioner. Do not take any herbal preparations if you are pregnant or breast-feeding without checking with your health adviser.

The list of herbs that are useful for medicinal use is phenomenal, and people will often develop an affinity with an individual herb or family. This can then become a constitutional cure, and one that it would be wise to keep in the medicine chest.

Experiment with the beneficial effects of herbal remedies when you next experience a minor health concern, and develop your own resource of useful remedies for yourself and your family.

Fresh herbs can be obtained from garden centres, supermarkets and grocers. Dried herbs can be found in many health-food shops and from specialist suppliers, along with prepared remedies in the form of tablets or tinctures.

Growing and Drying Your Own Herbs

Most herbs are easy to grow outdoors, or indoors on a sunny windowsill. Bringing them on from seed is a good way to ensure their quality, although it can take more than one season, especially with the more woody and slow-growing herbs like rosemary and eucalyptus. Buying a small plant from a good source will enable you to harvest some of the plant in the first year, whilst still being involved in the growing process. Most plants grow best in sandy soil that has good drainage and is not too rich, but refer to a good gardening book for individual advice. All plants respond well to lots of sunshine, and to being watered regularly. Remember that they are used to the world of outdoors, so even if you are growing them inside, take them out regularly so that they can feel their leaves being rustled by the wind, and experience the elements directly. Be sure to touch your plants as they are growing, and let the process enrich both you and them.

All growing things respond to love and care, so talk to your herbs as they are growing, and share some of the energy of your world with them. They also respond to music and pleasant sounds.

Pick any herbs for drying on a warm and sunny day. Show respect by carrying your intention to pick the plant in your mind as you approach it. If you get a feeling or a message that this is not a good day to pick, then listen to that. Approach this with an open mind, and you will soon discover how well we communicate with green things. If you feel that it is a good day to gather your herbs, pick as much as you want, but never all that is on the plant — leave something for the plant and/or another time. Lay your gatherings on some dry newspaper or kitchen towel, and put out in a sunny spot covered with a food frame or netting, or place in a very low oven overnight.

When dry, flake your herbs into a spotlessly clean pot or jar made of darkened glass (to protect its contents), and seal well. Sterilise your jar by pouring fast-boiling water over it, and then drying in a very low oven. Label and date your jar, and state whether the ingredients were home-grown or not. Store in a cool, dry place, and use within one year. The maximum potency will last for a little over three months on average, and after this the herb can be added to cooking or used in a slightly stronger ratio.

Making Tisanes and Infusions

Use a teaspoon of the dried herb or flower heads, and place in a dedicated teapot or jug. Cover with boiling water, and leave to infuse. The length of time will depend on your desired therapeutic effect and use, and on whether you are steeping flower heads or woodier parts of the plant. In general, steep leaves and flower-heads for up to 30 seconds before pouring, but leave them for much longer if it is a mild or delicate plant such as lemon balm, which requires longer to release its flavour. The fresh plant will require longer than the dried, and woody stems such as licorice can be left to stand for up to 5 minutes. Experiment for yourself with the taste and flavour of your choice of drinks.

If you are going to use the liquid for external application, e.g. for a compress or as a wash, or to add to bath-water, then make it double strength, and leave to stand for at least five minutes.

The following herbs are commonly available, and can often be grown in a garden, patio container or window-box for the additional benefits of their fresh, growing energy and to share in the beauty of their flowers.

Herb	Actions	How to Take
Aloe Vera	Stimulates the immune system and digestion. A strong wound healer and skin salve.	As a juice, or use the sap from a fresh leaf.
Borage	Stimulates adrenaline, promotes sweating, light sedative and very uplifting.	Grow the beautiful blue flowers, and add to salads and ice-cubes, take as a tea.

Herb	Actions	How to Take
Calendula	Speeds healing and soothes skin. Strong anti-inflammatory, has a strong affinity with the kidneys.	Steep the flowers to use as a wash, or to add to the bath-water. Take as a tea.
Camomile	Calming for nerves and digestion. Tonic for the stomach, and relieves fever.	Take the tea as a digestive after meals.
Echinacea	Powerful immune stimulant. Speeds circulation and cleanses the blood. Reduces inflammation and has strong anti-fungal and anti-bacterial properties.	Take as a tincture: 10 drops in a small glass of water once a day for three weeks, then take one week off. Or take the tea daily.
Feverfew	Anti-spasmodic pain reliever, useful for migraine sufferers.	Eat a sandwich of the fresh leaf, or take a strong tea daily. Can irritate sensitives.
Goldenseal	Fights infection and acts as a salve on the whole digestive system. Excellent to soothe inflammation and irritable bowel.	Dried root can be added to meals, or taken in tablet form.
Hawthorn	Cardiac tonic, improves peripheral circulation and will strengthen all smooth muscle.	Take a tea made from the berries or add to bath-water.

Herb	Actions	How to Take
Lemon Balm	Calming and relaxing with a gentle uplifting quality. Anti-viral, aids digestion and prevents flatulence.	Crush the fresh leaves and inhale deeply, or take as tea.
Saw Palmetto	Strong tonic. Inhibits prostate enlargement.	The berries can be in tablet form or as a tea or tincture.
Slippery Elm	Nutrient that relieves pain and soothes and protects the mucous membranes.	Take the dried bark in powder form added to meals, or mixed into a paste with apple juice and drunk before meals.
St John's Wort	Anti-depressant with strong wound-healing effects.	Grow for their beauty, and make the leaves and sunny yellow flowers into tea to drink daily. Make an oil for external use.
Wild Yam	Balances progesterone activity and is useful before and during the menopause. Anti-inflammatory.	Use a cream made of the root, and apply daily. Take the tincture to relieve cramping.

Flowers

These have been used for centuries to uplift the spirits and make us feel better. Flowers encourage us to share in their beauty, and can have a beneficial effect upon us just by being there. Aboriginal people and Native Americans have always worked with flowers as with all other aspects of Creation that can benefit us if we remain in balance with them.

Earlier this century, an English doctor, Edward Bach, began to refine the use of distilled flower essences, and these have since become widely available. He would gather the flowers and steep them in water for sunlight to maximise the extraction, and then distil this essence, preserving it with a drop of brandy. He maintained that there were several types or classes of illness or disharmony that the flowers could assist with, ranging from depression and loneliness to excess stoicism. He formulated the range of Bach Flower Remedies, and the composite Rescue Remedy which is so useful for all forms of distress from the pain of injury to the dread of a visit to the dentist, or exam nerves.

Nowadays there is an increasing interest in these gentle healers, and ranges of remedies from all parts of the world have been developed or refined. Some rely on locally available flowers; others use ocean flowers that are pan-global. As we remember our sense of one-ness with the rest of creation, it becomes easier to accept the gifts from these beautiful flowers, and many ranges of remedies are being developed that do not require the flowers to be picked or disturbed in any way. There are also those which do not use alcohol in their preparations, and this makes them more suitable for everyone.

Flower remedies all have a definite effect on the emotional level, and this is where their strength lies. They seem to have a softness which allows them to reach into our hearts and heal the wounds that lie there and in our emotions and feelings. These changes then have an impact on every other level of our life.

Bring the beauty of flowers into your life and into your world by growing them, and keeping them in and around your home. Discover for yourself those with which you feel most comfortable, allowing your own healing repertoire to grow as you begin to work with this gentle energy. There are some traditional affinities, such as roses representing love and enhancing feminine energy, but you will soon be able to discover your own favourites. Bring their energy further into your life by collecting any dew that gathers on their petals to add to your bath-water or place on your pulse points.

Add two drops of Dr Bach's Crab Apple flower remedy to soaking solution for a compress to treat skin complaints, and to relieve lower back pain and congestion.

The brand remedies can be used in the same way, applying them to the pulse points whenever they are desired. They will be absorbed through the skin very easily and quickly, and this is a sound choice for anyone not wishing to drink the remedy because of its alcohol content. The remedies can also be used in a soaking solution for any compress. Otherwise, take several drops either directly on to your tongue or in a small glass of water, several times a day. Make sure to take a dose early in the morning, and another before bed, and then as many times during the day as you can manage — ideally three-four. To simplify this, add several drops of the remedy to a small bottle of mineral water each morning, and keep in the fridge, taking a drink of it whenever you can. This also makes it easy to keep up your regular dose when travelling away from home.

Take one remedy at a time, or make a mix of those you feel drawn to, up to a maximum of five in any one blend. Each range will give full details of its remedies, and these can be found in a range of stores and health-food shops.

Although the Bach range is limited to European flowers, it is the most widely available, and the following is a sample of the conditions for which remedies are available under this brand. It is worth bearing in mind, however, that production has been taken over by a large company and is now mechanised.

The main categories are:

- fear
- uncertainty
- insufficient interest in present circumstances
- loneliness
- over-sensitivity to influences and ideas
- despondency or despair, and
- over-care for the welfare of others.

The remedies for fear include Rock Rose which is a wonderful steadier in extreme circumstances; Mimulus, useful for fear of worldly things; Cherry Plum for anxiety about becoming over-extended; Aspen for unexplained fears that are often kept secret; and Red Chestnut for those who pick up other people's emotions. Each main category contains a variety of remedies to help make assessment easier, although if you feel drawn to any individual remedy, trust your own intuition and take it, perhaps leaving until later an understanding of why it was the most suitable.

Perhaps the best known blend of the Dr Bach range is Rescue Remedy. This can be used in any number of situations, and is now also available in a cream. Apply this to burns for immediate relief, and to bruises and scrapes to soothe the area and aid resolution. This has a marked pain-relieving effect and speeds healing.

The following list is a guide to the range of flower remedies that is now available. Do not let the wide selection daunt you; rather let it comfort you in the knowledge that there is a flower remedy that will suit you from amongst this choice.

- Andreas Korte Essences come from Africa and the Amazon. They are made without picking the flowers, but by extracting the harmonic energy of their essence with the use of crystals.
- Bush Flower Essences and Living Essences come from Australia and build on the ancient lore of the aboriginal people, as do the New Perception Flower Essences which come from New Zealand.

- Bailey Essences, Findhorn Flower Essences, Green Man Tree Essences and Harebell Remedies are among the range that join the Bach Flower Remedies and come from the UK.
- Deva Flower Elixirs come from France.
- Himalayan Aditi, Himalayan Flower Enhancers and Himalayan Indian Tree and Flower Essences all come from India, and incorporate some of the traditional Ayurvedic teachings.
- Desert Alchemy Flower Essences, Pegasus Essences, Petite Fleur Essences and Perelandra Virginian Rose and Garden Essences are among the wide range that hail from the United States.
- Hawaiian Tropical Flower Essences build on the Polynesian understandings of life and harmony.
- Pacific Essences and Flower and Gem Remedies come from Canada.

More ranges are appearing as we begin to plumb the rich resource that flowers make available to us.

Essential Oils

These wonderfully aromatic oils are distilled or extracted from plants, herbs and flowers. They have almost universal applications around the home and for our ongoing health both in terms of supporting the immune system, and as fast-acting problem solvers. Their aroma is one of the most important aspects of this form of remedy, being able to reach the brain and be absorbed into the blood stream more quickly than just about any other type of cure. The use of essential oils has become popular as part of Aromatherapy Massage, when a blend of oils is applied to the body by a professional therapeutic massage practitioner. Any of the oils can be used in this way for self massage, or to work on friends and family members. They can also be used:

- to add to the bath
- to enhance the effects of a compress
- in skin and hair care
- to add to steam inhalations
- to perfume a room
- for neat applications directly on to the skin (only with great care and specificity, see below)

Essential oils are concentrated and very strong. They are needed in very small quantities to be effective. That means adding only 2–3 drops to a bath-full of warm water for a lovely soak, or two drops to a compress or bowl of boiled water for a steam inhalation. Apply them directly on to the skin on rare occasions, e.g. use lavender directly on to insect bites and stings, ti-tree oil on to verucae or blisters. When using in this way, apply using a cotton bud and make sure that the surrounding area is protected with a smear of Vaseline or oil. Never apply over an area of broken skin.

Not all essential oils that you buy are pure; sometimes they are already blended with oils and can therefore be used more liberally. Always check the labels before you use them. The price varies enormously depending upon how abundantly the herb grows and how easy it is to extract the oil. Jasmine and Rose are at the more expensive end of the market, but their strong, heady perfume goes a long way, and no more than one drop is ever needed at a time. More common herbs such as thyme and rosemary are less expensive. Essential oils are available from specialist suppliers, many chemists, and health-food shops. Store them in dark bottles that will protect them, and keep them in a cool place.

When using the oils, add to a base of carrier oil. This can be olive oil or anything from your kitchen, or a special blend of massage or dispersant oils. Choose from the range at your local chemist or health-food shop.

Do not use essential oils if you are pregnant or breast feeding without the advice of your natural healthcare practitioner. This is very important because some oils have a very strong effect on the system and can cross the placenta.

Essential oils are most often used individually for their therapeutic effects, and some of the most useful are in this table:

Essential Oil	Uses
Clary Sage	Warming and soothing. Good for chest, and to aid muscle relaxation. Has a strongly enhancing effect on dreams. Avoid alcohol when using, and do not drive or operate machinery immediately after use.

Essential Oil	Uses
Eucalyptus	A powerful decongestant that is excellent for clearing sinus complaints and for warming the chest area. Add a drop to a handkerchief for day-long use, and place a drop on the pillowslip at night to cure snoring.
Frankincense or Olibanum	A wonderfully soothing oil that will calm the nerves and deepen and relax the breath. Use in massage, or to perfume a room.
Geranium	This refreshing oil will balance the body and uplift the spirits. It has a wonderfully calming effect on the emotions, and can be added to the bath-water for a soak, or used in massage or to perfume a room.
Jasmine	A strong anti-depressant with a beautiful, evocative scent that lingers. Use in massage, add to the bath, and to scent a room.
Lavender	Balances the system, cools, and boosts overall immunity. Has strong antiseptic quality and can be applied carefully directly on to the site of bites and stings.
Ti-Tree	An incredible anti-viral, anti-bacterial, anti-fungal oil that comes from Australasia. Use to boost the immune system, added to a wash for the skin, or to bath-water, or to scent a room. Can also be applied directly with care to warts etc.

Scenting a Room

Essential oils can be used beyond the person for their special effects within a room or office.

- Use a few drops of thyme essential oil for protection when colds and flus are circulating, and this is especially useful for sore throats.
- Lemongrass has a powerful disinfectant quality, and a strong ability to ground and centre a person.
- Choose Rose for a bedroom or when needing to be uplifted.
- Rosemary makes a wonderful study aid, useful when needing to stimulate the memory.

There are many ways to spread these essential oils:

- Add two drops to a dry duster and use to wipe over radiator tops, light bulbs, and all areas that will heat up and diffuse the scent.
- Add two drops to a bowl of water and place over a radiator or other heat source, or in the summer place in front of an open window.
- Add two drops to a bowl of water, and soak a freshly-laundered tea towel in it. Wring out and drape within the room; over a radiator if possible.
- Add two drops to the small bowl of water over a specialist aromatherapy oil burner.
- Add a few drops to the rinsing water when washing curtains and loose covers.

Making an Individual Blend

Make a mixture of essential oils that is specific to you. This can be medicinal or purely aromatic. Follow your nose with this, and allow yourself to be guided towards those aromas which seem to reach you and please you. Check the therapeutic values of your chosen oils to help you decide how best to use them. You may choose a constitutional blend, for instance, during the colder weather to warm and hearten you. If you have a cold chest, and get sinus congestion, then eucalyptus would be a first choice, together with rosemary, thyme or geranium to lift your spirits. Keep this blend as long as you continue to respond to it, and use it all around you: burn it or use it to perfume your room, add two drops to your bath-water at least once a week, and carry a small bottle with you to use as an inhaler, either directly or by placing a few drops on a handkerchief.

If menstrual difficulties trouble you, then choose Howood, a powerful pelvic decongestant, Rose for its effect as a uterine tonic, and Clary Sage or Sandalwood to warm and comfort you.

These oils can also be used as a perfume that will have good therapeutic effects. Bear the medicinal values in mind before you decide on your final blend, but look to a different form of classification if a perfume is your primary choice.

All Essential Oils can be described as giving off an aroma that is:

- Woody — like cedarwood or pine;
- Herbaceous — like marjoram or clary sage;

- Citrus — like bergamot and lemon;
- Floral — like rose and geranium;
- Resinous — like olibanum and jasmine;
- Spicy — like ginger and black pepper.

Traditionally, oils blend best with other oils from the same grouping, and those from neighbouring groups, so in theory, cedarwood and pine would work well together, and would blend well with clary sage or marjoram.

A well rounded perfume, though, will have three important elements: a top note that is light and fresh, and is often the first scent that you will be able to identify; a middle note that is longer lasting and carries the main force of the scent; and a base note that is usually richer and heavier, and lingers longest of all.

Experiment for yourself with these oil blends, and do not be surprised if you discover that those oils you chose purely for their scent turn out to have just the therapeutic effects that you need.

Tissue Salts

These are a remarkable range of minerals in a form that the body can assimilate most easily. The minerals are formed into salts and tableted with lactose, so they are suitable for everyone (except those with a marked lactose intolerance). They are safe to use and fast acting, which makes them suitable for treating a wide range of concerns, and especially appropriate for acute conditions or those which come on suddenly. They also work extremely effectively to treat deep-seated or long-term complaints, because they directly address any imbalance at its root.

Tissue salts can be taken in response to immediate health concerns, as seasonal remedies, or as constitutional strengtheners. Some of the symptoms of ill health will reflect more deep-seated imbalances which will profit from longer term treatment.

There are twelve individual or simple tissue salts, and these have been formulated into eighteen additional or compound remedies. You can take your own mixture of simple remedies, according to your symptom picture and why you are taking them, or take a compound remedy specifically for your complaint. Some remedies work most effectively when alternated with another, or when taken with one or more Tissue Salts that will enhance their action.

Tissue salts can be bought from your chemist or health food shop in small pots that contain dozens of the tiny lactose tablets. Take them as directed on the pot, and decant them into the lid before putting them into your mouth — do not touch them with your hands. This will reduce the risk of spoiling the delicate balance of the tablet with any contaminant that you may have on your hands. The tablets are designed to dissolve on your tongue, leaving a slightly sweet taste in your mouth. They enter the blood stream very quickly, and effects can often be felt straight away.

Trained practitioners will often use Tissue Salts as part of a complex nutritional plan, but they are totally suitable for home use, and prove an effective answer to a range of everyday health concerns for all the family.

Take the tablets for as long as symptoms persist. Leave at least 20 minutes between having foods or strong flavoured drinks (e.g. coffee, peppermint tea) or brushing your teeth, and taking the tablets. Monitor the changes that you are experiencing, and note for yourself which remedies work best. For ongoing concerns, consider taking the tissue salts for up to three weeks at a time. When using to treat cyclic complaints, such as menstrual cramping, expect to see some changes straight away, but anticipate repeating the treatment dosage with subsequent periods. On occasion, the initial response to taking the Tissue Salts will be an aggravation or worsening of the symptoms. Take this as a good sign — meaning that you have hit the nail on the head so to speak, and continue with subsequent doses. Any worsening is usually very quick to pass and is followed by a great relief of the whole symptom picture.

The full range of Tissue Salts is shown below. Each mineral is called by its Latin name, and known by its abbreviated form:

Tissue Salt	Uses
Calc. Fluor. (Calcium Fluoride)	Useful builder of elastic tissue. Good for treating muscular weakness, poor circulation and dental decay. An excellent wound healer.
Calc. Phos. (Calcium Phosphate)	Vital to the formation of new blood cells. Excellent treatment for low-energy complaints and when convalescing.
Calc. Sulph. (Calcium Sulphate)	Purifies the blood and enhances a number of processes within the body. Cleanses the skin.

Tissue Salt	Uses
Ferr. Phos. (Iron Phosphate)	Increases oxygen uptake and carriage in the blood. Aids circulation, energy levels, mental activity and mobility. An excellent choice of tonic for older people.
Kali. Mur. (Potassium Chloride)	Conditions the blood. Useful to treat all forms of congestion and a variety of mucus conditions.
Kali. Phos. (Potassium Phosphate)	Nerve nutrient. Excellent in treating nervous complaints, also good with depression and for tension and nervous headaches.
Kali.Sulph. (Potassium Sulphate)	Oxygenates all tissue cells. A useful tissue salt to alternate with others. Shows general improvements in the skin, hair and nails.
Mag. Phos. (Magnesium Phosphate)	A powerful anti-spasmodic. Will fight cramps, shooting pains and flatulence. Useful for painful periods and also for toothache.
Nat. Mur. (Sodium Chloride)	Ensures good water distribution throughout the body. A strong seasonal remedy for autumn and winter, and to relieve the runny nose of colds and allergic reactions.
Nat. Phos. (Sodium Phosphate)	Neutralises acidity. Useful for rheumatic and arthritic complaints, and will soothe stomach complaints and relieve acid indigestion.

Tissue Salt	Uses
Nat. Sulph. (Sodium Sulphate)	Eliminates excess water from the system, and will help regulate all congestive concerns, from flu to water-retention, swellings and biliousness.
Silica (Silicic Oxide)	Cleansing and eliminative. Will regulate the menstrual cycle as well as improving bowel function and cleansing the skin.

You can mix three or more simple remedies together to achieve a good balanced treatment for your individual concerns. Consider, too, alternating one or two remedies that seem to be appropriate or that will work in harmony together.

> Some Tissue Salts can be used externally: crush a few tablets of Ferr. Phos between very clean fingers and rub them into any cleaned cut or graze to speed healing.

Many health complaints are common to a number of people, and will tend to be a reflection of an imbalance in a particular Tissue Salt or combination of Tissue Salts, and to this end, a range of composite remedies has been formulated. These can be useful if you recognise your health concerns from the following list, and will save you the trouble of mixing your own simple remedies together.

Neuralgia and allied conditions — Combination A
Convalescence, and as a general energy-booster — Combination B

Acidity and heartburn — Combination C
Skin complaints — D
Flatulence, colic and indigestion — E
Nervous headaches and migraines — F
Backache and piles — G
Hay fever and other allergic responses — H
Muscle Pain — I
Colds, coughs and chestiness — J (This is a wonderful seasonal remedy for autumn and winter)
Brittle nails and hair loss — K
Poor circulation — L
Rheumatism — M
Cramps (including period pains) — N
Aching feet and legs — P
Catarrh and sinus congestion — Q
Infant's teething pains — R
Nausea, stomach upsets and headaches — S (a good seasonal remedy for summer).

Nutritional Supplements

Vitamins and minerals are the most common nutritional supplements that we take, although this category also includes trace elements, bioflavonoids and other food-related supplements, and some herb and plant extracts that are best taken in tablet or supplement form.

All of us who are over 35 years old, live more than a mile from the sea and experience any form of stress or change in our lives, need to consider nutritional supplements. They can address long term dietary deficiency, augment a poor diet, and treat specific symptoms.

> Tinnitus is a debilitating condition characterised by continuous ringing or noise in the ears. Causes can range from an excess of ear wax to trauma, or poor circulation, and it can also occur in response to loud music and Zinc deficiency. Consider supplementing with 60–90 mg of a form of Zinc that includes copper for three weeks, and take Ginkgo biloba as a tea or a supplement daily during that time. The symptoms may also respond to cranio-sacral therapy, so ask your practitioner for further information about this specialist form of bodywork.

Individual vitamins and minerals are best prescribed by your practitioner, who will know your full nutritional status and be best placed to advise you with specific regard to your own needs. There are a few exceptions to this, including Vitamin C, the hero of the immune system and champion of the fight against the common cold. This vitamin has a marked protective effect in the body, and most of us in the West could profit from having a lot more circulating Vitamin C in our system than we do. It is involved in all manner of physical activities from wound healing to reproduction, and so many of our modern lifestyle activities deplete the body of this valuable nutrient. Ageing, smoking, drinking alcohol, experiencing stress and encountering viruses and bacteria all rob the body of Vitamin C. Take a low dose Vitamin C supplement several times a day for the best effect.

Choose a product that is 250–500 mg and has no flavourings, colourings, etc. Rosehip is a good source, and the only addition you would expect to see to the Vitamin itself is bioflavonoids, naturally occurring substances which assist in its absorption.

Always take Vitamin C with or immediately after some food for maximum absorption and safety. Take 1g a day as a maintenance dose throughout times of additional stress, and double that amount to face a health crisis. Do not take it at all the rest of the time. Take care when you discontinue taking your Vitamin C supplement: do not stop suddenly, but reduce your dose by half, then take every other dose, and phase it out slowly over anything up to one month.

The range of B Vitamins, or B-Complex, are useful stress busters, and can also be taken when the body is under pressure and in need of additional support. Never take individual B Vitamins without the advice of your natural healthcare practitioner. Always choose a balanced B Complex from a good supplier which will contain the full range of B Vitamins.

Vitamin E is a useful supplement to have in the home for external application. This is invaluable for skin healing and to treat minor burns once they have cooled. It can also be applied to stretch marks or scar tissue, and can be used routinely on the face in place of moisturiser. The capsules are easy to pierce with a pin, and you can apply them straight away. The oil is thick and heavy, and you need very little to have a positive effect.

Calcium is a mineral that is much under the spotlight because of its role in the maintenance of healthy teeth and bones, and the prevention of osteoporosis. It is a very immediate answer to dental caries and fractures. This mineral works together with a range of others to ensure maximum uptake in the body, so look for a Calcium-Magnesium supplement with Boron if you feel you are in need of additional calcium. Do not take this for more than one month without consulting a natural healthcare practitioner.

There are times when we all need additional support, and this is when a multiple supplement could be most useful. I would certainly recommend taking one at the change of season, when experiencing high stress, embarking on a new exercise or dietary plan, and if noticing low energy levels. They can also be very useful while travelling and when undertaking any new direction in life. Take them for as short a time as you can, shifting the focus back on to gaining the nutrients that you need from your diet and your lifestyle. Choose your time to stop taking them, however, and ease them out gently: reduce your dose by half, and take them every other day over a period of about two–three weeks to enable your body to get used to the change.

Seek out a good supplement supplier, or ask your practitioner for their recommendation (or see the Resource section, page 220). The quality of the product is most important, and wherever possible you will want to pay as much attention to the type, freshness and source of your supplements as you would to the food you eat. Most serious nutritional suppliers will offer a range of balanced multi-vitamin and mineral formulae. To help with your choice, there is a standard internationally recognised minimum level of each nutrient that is required every day for ongoing health. This is known as the Recommended Daily

Allowance or RDA. It is laughably small, so make sure that the product you choose is supplying at least the RDA across the range of nutrients it provides.

Vitamin/Mineral	RDA
A	2,500IU (International Units)
B Complex:	
B1 Thiamine	10 mg
B2 Riboflavin	5 mg
B3 Niacin	10 mg
B5 Pantoghenic Acid	not yet agreed
B6 Pyridoxine	2 mg
B12 Cyanocobalamin	50 mcg
Biotin	150-300 mcg
Choline	650 mg *(This is a maximum dose)
Inositol	Not yet agreed. Likely to be around 1,000 mg
Folic Acid	0.4 mg
Para Amino Benzoic Acid (PABA)	Not yet agreed. Likely to be around 100 mg
Vitamin C	30 mg
Vitamin D Cholecalciferol	100IU
Vitamin E Tocopherol	30IU
Calcium	500 mg
Copper	less than 1 mg
Iodine	200 mcg

Vitamin/Mineral	RDA
Iron	Completely variable — a woman generally loses 15-30 mg with each menstrual period
Magnesium	150-450 mg
Manganese	2 mg
Phosphorus	1.5-2 mg
Potassium	2-4 mg
Selenium	150 mcg
Sodium	2 mg
Zinc	15 mg. Long term supplementation with zinc is not advised, because it can have a depleting effect upon the immune system.

Most important of all is that you read the label, and do not choose any product that contains sugar, sucrose, flavourings, colourings, preservatives, or any of the range of chemical additives and fillers that you would not find acceptable in your food. The ingredients list on supplement bottles is the same as in foodstuffs in that it presents the major ingredients first, so if you choose a Vitamin C supplement that lists sugar or sweetener, colouring, flavouring and preservatives before it lists the Vitamin C, then you would do better to suck on a jelly bean — it will be considerably cheaper, and you will not be fooling yourself into thinking that you are taking anything good into your body.

Beyond vitamin and mineral supplements, there is a variety of herbal and other remedies that are most useful when taken as nutritional aids. Some of the more commonly available include:

- Ginko Bilboa — a tablet made from the nut of the most ancient tree on earth. It increases the flow of blood to the brain and reduces the ageing of tissues.
- Lecithin — A naturally-occurring substance involved in fat transportation within the body. Available as granules, capsules or in liquid form.
- Spirulina — A blue-green alga which is high in protein and has a strong cleansing effect on the body. A rare source of Vitamin B12. Available in tablets.
- Silymarine — Extract of the Milk Thistle Herb. This is a powerful cleanser and supports liver function, improves the skin, and will treat gall-bladder and biliary complaints.
- Pycnogenol — A powerful antioxidant, extract of the Pine tree.
- Psyllium Husks — Available in powder or capsule form to increase intestinal bulk and cleanse the bowel.
- Charcoal — Choose a naturally activated brand and take as directed on the pot to relieve gas and a range of digestive complaints. Also useful to take when facing dental work or other minor procedures, because Charcoal absorbs the substances it finds in the stomach and beyond, neutralising them and enabling them to be passed out of the system. Take only when necessary, because it also absorbs nutrients, and takes them out of the system with it.

- Garlic and ginger are among the extensive range of more common medicinals that can also be taken in tablet or capsule form to enable a larger dose that is easier to fit into more lifestyle situations.

All these nutritional aids are available from specialist suppliers, many chemists, and health food shops. Always consider your need carefully before selecting any nutritional supplement, and seek professional advice if you are not sure as to your own individual requirements.

Treat these remedies as gifts, and use them wisely, taking care not to abuse them or take them for granted because that would be to dishonour the giver. Let them bring you assistance, support and encouragement when you need their special qualities, but endeavour not to use them as a crutch to enable continued bad health habits. Allow their presence to reassure you that whatever your needs, there is a specially formulated remedy that is available to meet your own individual prescription.

Chapter 7

THE KITCHEN PHARMACY

Beyond the foods and drinks that can influence your health, there is a range of home remedies that live in your kitchen, or can be made there. There is something quite wonderful about preparing your own cures, and knowing that you have incorporated all the best energies and ingredients in order to make something that will meet your personal needs.

Always choose the purest and best whenever you are making your own remedies, or even when employing a simple measure like applying fresh lemon juice or a spoonful of honey. Select things that are naturally or organically grown, and where possible pick fresh produce for yourself. This may encourage you to grow some of your own herbs and flowers, so you will have a whole variety of health-enhancing effects. There is always space for some of your favourite or most useful plants, whether you have a garden or are relying on patio tubs, window boxes or just the kitchen window-sill.

The following list includes some of my own favourites, and you may already know of remedies, scents and plants that suit you:

Plant	Special Qualities and Applications
Lavender	Easy to grow, and a wonderful scent to perfume any area. Crush a flower directly on to an insect bite or sting for instant relief. Add the plant to bath water for a cooling and soothing energy lift.
Marigolds	These beautiful flowers will bloom early and bring a wash of strong colour to early spring. Add the flowers to salads and sandwiches for a vitamin-enriched treat. Dry the flowers and steep them in water to make a skin-cleansing tonic.
Roses	Their wonderfully evocative scent has a strong affinity with the feminine, and is a useful uterine tonic. Their beauty always lifts the heart, and they can be cut and brought indoors to perfume any room. Add rose petals to salads for a wonderfully fragrant garnish, and make into a jam for an old-fashioned treat that is deliciously cooling and settling for the digestion.
Red Sage	A beautiful plant whose leaves can be added to cooking for their curative values. Make red sage tea and drink a small cupful every day when there is a risk of coughs and colds. Use as a gargle to relieve sore and dry throats and ease bronchitis. Can also be made into a poultice (see below) as a treatment for a stiff neck. Burn dried sage to cleanse an area and instil a spiritual sense.

Plant	Special Qualities and Applications
Thyme	This powerfully-scented plant is a reliable ally as a cleanser and healer. Keep some sprigs indoors, and use to antidote any airborne germs. Add to meals for its antiseptic qualities — especially useful when eating meat. Crumble the leaves into a bowl and treat as a pot-pourri to lend its disinfectant qualities to a sick-room, bathroom, or any other part of the home or work place.

Many of the items in your kitchen cupboards can be used to great effect as first-aid cures and to treat ongoing minor health concerns. During the summer months, bicarbonate of soda and vinegar are tremendously useful to keep around, especially when the weather becomes warmer and you are spending more time out of doors. Use bicarbonate of soda to relieve the pain of bee stings, and dab wasp stings with vinegar.

Vinegar is a wonderful store-cupboard cure-all that will relieve sunburn and has a host of other applications. Drink a glass of warm water every morning to which a tablespoon of apple cider vinegar has been added, and sweeten to taste with a little honey if necessary for you. This has a strong alkalinising effect on the system and will relieve acid complaints and the joint soreness of arthritis. Put a capful of apple cider vinegar in a tall glass of warm water to use as a mouthwash whenever you have ulcers, or if is cold and flu season. Use a capful in the bath water as an on-going protective measure for women. Apple cider vinegar can be used in a stronger preparation to treat vaginal thrush directly: Add a cupful to the bath water, and make sure to swish the water around fully before sitting in. Avoid using soap, and 'wash' the whole area between your legs with the bath water. If the thrush proves stubborn, douche with a solution made from one capful of the vinegar in a gallon of warm water.

Yoghurt is a useful soother and will bring instant relief to a range of irritable skin conditions. Apply as cold as you can bear, and allow the coolness of the treatment to be as much of a balm as the yoghurt itself. This can be applied to a feminine pad and will bring great relief if there is thrush or any similar complaint. Eat live yoghurt to help the system recover from diarrhoea or other digestive upsets, and always take some after a course of antibiotic treatment to repopulate the gut with beneficial bacteria.

Another great kitchen medicine is the lemon. This has a myriad uses. Always choose a naturally or organically grown lemon, or, at the very least, one that has not been waxed. These are becoming much more widely available, and many supermarkets now stock them. Add a slice of lemon and a good squeeze of the fresh juice to a glass of warm water for an early morning drink that will cut through any mucus congestion and prove an effective detox. Add a good squeeze of the juice to a small glass of warm water for an instant fix of Vitamin C, and take as often as you like. This is also a great cleanser if you have been eating a lot of fatty foods and feel congested or stuck. Apply a few drops of fresh lemon juice directly on to a mouth ulcer or a cold sore for a speedy cure. It does sting, but the direct hit of Vitamin C, fruit acid, and essential oil of lemon mean that the condition will disappear very quickly. Use this three to five times a day until no longer needed. Often this will clean up any problem within about two days.

A squeeze of fresh lemon juice is also a good cure for warts. Apply directly on to the wart and then expose the area to sunlight. The best kitchen cure for warts, though, is strangely old-fashioned: Rub the affected area with the cut surface of a potato, and then bury the potato. The wart will disappear as the potato rots away. This works — I have used it myself, and with my patients, who are often sceptical, but it is the most effective and consistent miracle.

During the summer, protecting yourself when out of doors is very important and becoming more so as we continue to damage this planet's own protective layers. If you experience any degree of sunburn, add a cupful of vinegar to a basin of warm water, and lightly sponge the whole of the affected area. This wash will relieve much of the heat and sting of the burn. This will usually reduce the risk of blisters, but if they do occur, cover with honey and hold in place with a light gauze. Replace the honey as often as you can — the skin will usually seem to drink it in.

Honey is a great healer, and can be used to speed the skin's own healing efforts, as well as to relieve the pain of burns and blistering. Cover any minor burn with a thick paste of honey and you can almost watch it begin to recover. This is also an effective remedy to use on old scars. Honey works very effectively to smother any yeast or fungal infections, and regular applications to any form of skin trouble are usually wholly beneficial.

An amazing cure for minor burns is to immerse the area in warm water. This seems to draw out the pain quite dramatically and can feel very intense, but once the wave of heat has subsided there is rarely any discomfort left, and the area is normally left clear and blister-free. The easiest way to do this is to fill the sink or basin with water that is quite hot, but certainly not going to burn. Immerse the hand or other area in the water, and keep it there — this is the difficult part because a wave of burning sensation rises quite quickly, but bear with it and within minutes the area will be feeling fine again.

Athlete's foot is a minor but extremely irritating complaint that can prove surprisingly stubborn. There are a number of natural cures and remedies that can all be equally effective, depending on the cause of the complaint. It can simply be a question of feet needing to breathe, rather than being cooped up inside the synthetic material of stockings or socks and shoes for up to eighteen hours every day. Letting your feet spend some time in the open is a good idea for ongoing health anyway, so is recommended whatever your state of health. The fungus growth can be treated directly with regular applications of Ti-Tree essential oil, and by being smothered in honey overnight. Achieve this by applying liberal amounts of thick, set honey to your feet after bathing and carefully drying them, and then covering with a pair of thin socks. Repeat this every night for a week, and you will be able to see the effects. If the condition is particularly stubborn, or has lasted for a long time, repeat the honey application in the mornings, although this is a little less easy. Peeing on your feet is a good precautionary measure that will keep athlete's foot at bay if there has been a problem in the past. There is often a dietary connection too, and it is recommended that you review the amount of yeast and sugar, wheat and cow's dairy foods that you are eating.

Epsom Salts are a useful store-cupboard cure, being easy to apply and a speedy solution to all manner of aches and pains. Add 1 lb of Epsom Salts to a hot bath, and soak for as long as you can to relieve any muscle strain. Do not do this if you have any heart problems. Otherwise, it is wonderfully soothing and relaxing, and works to relieve back-ache, menstrual cramps and minor sporting injuries. For a more localised effect, add a handful of the Salts to a basin of hot water. Soak a freshly-laundered tea-towel in the solution and then wring out and apply, as hot as you can bear, to the affected area. Reapply as soon as the cloth cools. This is a great instant remedy for low back pain, and works really well as a poultice for the liver or spleen (see below.) Use a handful of Epsom Salts in a foot bath of warm water if you have been on your feet all day, and once the water has cooled, lie down with your feet elevated above the level of your heart (i.e. propped up on cushions), for ten minutes.

Treat earache and jaw pain by heating a tray of sea salt in the oven, and carefully decanting into a cotton pocket, or a freshly laundered handkerchief that you can fold over and secure. Hold this in place over the painful side of the face, and lie down on it for comfort. This can be replaced once the salt cools, but it will hold its warmth for some time. This is tremendously soothing, and will often draw out any infection.

Foot baths are an easy way to treat the whole body. Add a teaspoon of mustard powder to a basin full of warm water and soak your feet until the water cools. This is a great cold remedy, and will feel as though it is drawing any congestion and cold right down through your body and out into the water. This is also very warming, and by adding a little extra mustard powder you can heat up your system after a chill. This is a very good way to clear any sinus congestion too.

Add some sprigs of fresh lavender to a basin full of tepid water and soak your feet in it to cool and soothe away any tiredness on a hot day. This will also relieve any mild headache that is heat-related, and can have a positive effect on the congestion that comes from hay-fever and other allergies.

Make a bread poultice to draw out any infection surrounding a boil or skin abrasion. Soak some crustless bread in warm water for five minutes, and then wring out well. Apply to the area, and wrap in place with any form of bandage, sock or freshly-laundered tea-towel or handkerchief. Check the condition of the area every few hours, and replace the poultice each time. Continue to use for up to three days if there is a good response, and the area should be healed within that time.

Use salt to treat your whole body, enriching the condition of your skin and sloughing off dead skin cells that interfere with elimination: Take a handful of coarse sea-salt and add to a small basin of warm water so that a sort of slush develops. Use this to treat your whole body, or just isolated parts. Spread the slush on, and rub in as vigorously as you can, taking care not to cause yourself any discomfort. Rub the covered area with your hands for a few moments, and you will feel the action of the salt cleansing and drawing impurities out of your skin. Rinse off with warm water, and dry with a soft towel. Leave your skin to breathe for a while before deciding whether you need to moisturise it — twenty minutes or so will allow the skin to recover sufficiently from this salt bath.

Natural First Aid

The garlic, ginger and raw ingredients from your kitchen will often be all that you need to resolve minor health complaints. Keeping a supply of herbal infusions, infused oils and syrups will ensure that you have to hand a range of remedies that you can trust. Among those everyday ingredients that are invaluable:

- Garlic — rub a clove on to broken skin to disinfect, and relieve painful spots and corns.
- Aloe — grow the plant and use the sap from a fresh leaf to soothe minor burns, sunburns, and any skin irritation.
- Onion — place a fresh slice on insect stings, nettle rash, hives or urticaria for instant relief.
- Crystallised ginger — chew a small piece to ease nausea and prevent travel sickness.

- Propolis — available from bee-keepers and the health-food shop; a powerful nutritional aid.

Make a ginger poultice to relieve all manner of ills depending on where you place it. Ginger will warm the liver and assist in detoxifying the system and improving the efficiency of the gall bladder if you place the compress over it (on your right side, at the bottom of your rib cage). Use the compress to soothe the pain of a dental abscess and it will often cure it, and also to relieve headaches. Place two litres of water in a large saucepan that isn't aluminium or non-stick and add 8oz of freshly grated ginger root in a muslin bag. Bring to the boil, and place two freshly-laundered tea towels in the pot. Remove from the boil and simmer. Take one of the tea-towels out of the water very carefully, and wring out. Smear the area where you will place the compress with a little oil or Vaseline, and put the compress on top, wrapping it with a towel or similar to hold it in place. Replace it in the pot once it has cooled, and use the other tea-towel. Maintain the compress for about thirty minutes, or until relief is felt.

You can keep the pot of ginger water and the cloths to boil up and use on a second or third day, but after that it should be discarded. Make sure that you top up the water level each day so that the compress does not become too strong.

Making and Using Remedies

Whenever you are making a remedy, endeavour to include as many positive and beneficial aspects and energies as you possibly can. Incorporate some of the moon's magnificent magnetism by allowing it to guide your choice of timing — prepare those cures that will add something to the body when the moon is growing, and those that will remove something or rid the body of it when the moon is waning. Your cures can be prepared in the light of the sun, but bear in mind the phase of the moon in its monthly cycle of change.

Ensure that the place where you will be effecting your apothecarial magic is as clean and clear as possible. Burn some dried sage to cleanse the area, or open the windows and doors and allow the wind to clear out any negative energy and bring in all that is good. Check out your own humour on the day; do not endeavour to make your remedies and cures when you are feeling cross, over-tired, or sad and emotional. Similarly, choose a day that is bright and sunny, because the energy of the day will become part of your remedy.

- Endeavour to collect the ingredients for your cures yourself, and always choose the freshest and the best.
- Make sure that you have good containers for your cures, and sterilise them where appropriate. You can do this very simply by pouring fast-boiling water over them, and then drying slowly in a low oven.
- Label everything that you make, together with a date. It may be obvious now, but if the bottle or packet is moved, or when you have more of them, it can become very confusing indeed.

Remedies to Use Now

Infusions

A tea is one of the quickest and easiest ways to take a herb or flower, and the infusion can also form the basis of any physical application by providing a medium in which to soak a freshly-laundered handkerchief or tea-towel. Place one large teaspoon of dried herb, or two tablespoons of fresh herb into a dedicated teapot, and cover with water which has just come off the boil. Place the lid on and leave to stand for the time directed, usually 30 seconds to two minutes for internal use, and five minutes to one hour for external applications.

Use fresh leaves of lemon balm to fill the teapot and give you a calming, soothing and refreshing drink on a hot day. Prepare a double-strength infusion of red sage leaves and soak a freshly-laundered handkerchief in it. Wring out and wrap around the neck, covering with a towel, and go to bed for a speedy recovery from throat infections, neck pain and light coughs.

Decoctions

This is a way to extract the goodness from the bark or roots of a herb and is also used with some berries. This generally involves steeping and boiling the substance to encourage it to release its medicinal values. The herb bark should be crushed and placed in a pan, roots need to be washed and chopped or grated, and berries simply crushed. Place 1 oz of the herb in a saucepan that isn't aluminium or non-stick. Add 1 litre of cold water, and bring this to the boil. Simmer gently with the lid on until the liquid has reduced by about half, then remove from the heat and leave to stand and cool. Strain off the liquid and use the remaining plant material for the compost heap.

Make a strong decoction with camomile flowers, using 8 oz in a gallon of water. Soak them overnight in the water before boiling. Once prepared, pour the liquid straight into a bath full of warm water. Soak in this with the level of the water up over your kidneys to encourage speedy healing of pelvic inflammations and any skin complaints.

Poultices

These are made with crushed or chopped herbs that are heated and applied directly to the skin. They will soothe the area and tend to draw out any poisons. Place the herbs on a piece of cloth or a freshly-laundered handkerchief or tea-towel. Tie or fold the edges so that the herb is held safely, and immerse in boiling water until it is all soft and mushy. Squeeze out the water, and apply the poultice to the skin as hot as it can be borne. Hold in place by wrapping round with a freshly-laundered towel or cloth.

Use a whole, fresh cabbage leaf to cover a boil and draw it out. Place directly into boiling water for only a matter of seconds before applying as hot as can be borne to the skin, which has first been covered with a thin film of oil or Vaseline.

Compress

This is traditionally a cold application, and in its simplest form can mean crushing something directly on to the skin. When you bruise a dock leaf and press it on to a nettle sting you are using it as a compress. The easiest way to use a compress is to soak a freshly-laundered tea-towel or handkerchief in a herbal infusion, wring it out and apply it to the skin. If the soaking liquid has needed to be heated to release its medicinal qualities, then soak the cloth in the warm liquid.

Hold a cloth under the cold tap for the simplest compress that will bring relief to a headache or to neck pain and congestion.

Steam Inhalations

An old steam inhalation is often the easiest way to directly influence the skin of the face and neck, the mucous membranes and the chest. Add freshly-boiled water to a large bowl and cover with a freshly-laundered towel. Place your head in underneath the towel, and breathe in the steam for as long as you can bear. Come out of the 'tent' when you need some fresh air, but keep the bowl covered to retain the heat and the steam.

Add some freshly crushed thyme or rosemary leaves to the water for a fast-acting sinus decongestant.

Remedies to Keep

TINCTURES

This is a way of keeping a herb for a long time. The dried or fresh herb is steeped in a mixture of alcohol and water, and this extracts the plant's active ingredients and allows the preparation to be kept for up to a year. Use vodka or rubbing alcohol, and combine about 1 oz of the crushed or powdered herb with 2 pints of the alcohol and 4 pints of water. Store in an airtight container in a warm place, and shake the bottle every day for three to four weeks. The tincture should then be ready.

Not everybody chooses to take alcohol, but this makes an excellent application for those who do not want to drink it.

INFUSED OILS

Herbs release their properties into the oil which can then be used in massage blends, creams and ointments. The greater the proportion of herb, the stronger the effect of the mixture. Put 2 oz of crushed herb into a glass jar. Add 2 pints of olive or other vegetable oil, and 1 tablespoon of wine vinegar. Leave the jar in a warm place and shake the bottle every day for 2 weeks. Strain the oil, and add more fresh herbs, then continue to shake the bottle every day for another four to five weeks. The oil should then be ready.

Make an oil blend using sunflower oil and fresh St John's Wort. This is a light and cheery flower that will bring speedy healing to all skin complaints, and also has marked anti-depressant actions — useful whenever there is injury or discomfort.

Syrups

These are very pleasant and make for an easy way to take one's medicine. Pour 12 cups of boiling water on 3 oz of crushed herbs and leave to cool. Strain, and warm the liquid, adding 2 cups of sugar, and stirring until it is dissolved. Bring to the boil, and simmer gently until it reaches a thick, syrupy consistency. Cool slightly, then pour into a dark glass jar or bottle and label. Use a cork rather than a screw top because syrups often ferment and screw-top jars and bottles can explode.

Alternatively, heat a standard infusion or decoction in the saucepan, add honey or sugar to taste and then stir constantly until dissolved.

Add thyme honey to sweeten your syrup and disinfect the throat and lungs, and heather honey to strengthen the urinary system. Choose clover and orange blossom honeys to further soothe coughs and sore throats. Flavour your syrups with vanilla, licorice or aniseed to enhance the digestion and improve the taste still further. Take a teaspoon at a time and give children half the dose.

Body Packs

This is a wonderfully effective way to treat the body, and can be used on the whole trunk, or on isolated parts of the body such as the chest or neck.

For a neck pack, wet a freshly-laundered cotton handkerchief or strip of cotton cloth in cold water. Wring it out well and wrap around the neck. Cover this completely with a thick towel, and go to bed. Leave overnight if possible. This is an effective remedy for neck pain, sore throats and swollen glands. Enhance the effect by soaking in a cold infusion of red sage.

A chest pack is useful whenever there is the threat of bronchial involvement after a cold or flu. It will also help any digestive problems, and is generally warming and comforting. Wet a freshly-laundered tea-towel or cloth in cold water, and wring out well. Place on the chest in one layer, and then cover immediately with a thick towel, and wrap the body around in a downy, quilt or blankets. As before, retire to bed and leave the pack in place overnight if possible. The body should soon warm up, and the layer of cold cotton will warm and dry quite quickly. This is a very useful treatment for children, who will usually enjoy being packed up so warm and snug. If you are using this to treat a child, check that the cotton is in fact warm and dry by slipping your hand down inside the wrapping after one hour. If it is still wet or cold after that much time, unwrap the child, and warm him or her up. Consult your practitioner for an alternative remedy that will suit better.

Whole body packs are used to stave off colds and coughs, and at the first sign of flu. They will reduce a mild fever, and help with any muscle soreness or stiffness. The easiest way to do this is to line up a cotton vest, a cotton T-shirt and a cotton jumper, and have a downy, quilt or blankets to hand. Wet the cotton vest in cold water and wring it out well. Take a deep breath, and put it on. Then immediately put on the dry T-shirt and the jumper. Lie down, wrapped up well in the covers, and stay packed overnight if possible. If you have someone to help you, you can do this with two freshly-laundered tea towels, lying down on top of one, and having the other placed over your chest, and then being wrapped around snugly with a large towel, followed by the layers of quilt or blankets. Sleep is usually blissful when you are wrapped up in the security of a warm body pack.

Any of these measures can be repeated every three days, or once a week for children.

Smaller body parts can be treated this way with great success, e.g. soak a pair of cotton socks in cold water and wring them out well. Put on just before going to bed for an excellent night's sleep. This works very well for infants.

For the Home

Make a pot-pourri to scent your rooms naturally and enhance the therapeutic effects of any remedy. This is a mixture of sweet-smelling materials that is based on dried flower petals to which have been added aromatic herb seeds and spices, and occasionally a drop or two of essential oils.

Dry your own petals and leaves if you can, because this will ensure the highest quality and involve you in the entire process. Otherwise you can buy them from specialist suppliers and from some chemists and health food shops. Rose petals make a strong base, and will impart their subtle aroma in a most beautiful way within your home. Add dried sage, bay, lemon balm, peppermint, bergamot, rosemary, violets, jasmine, lavender and pinks from the summer flowering plants. Mix these together with a little common salt, and add some crushed coriander for a cooling but evocative scent; cloves for a warmer mix, or any from the range of cinnamon, nutmeg, vanilla, allspice or any individual aroma you especially like or respond well to.

Place the dried mixture in open bowls around the house, and turn them each time you pass to release more of the fragrance.

Herb cushions are another lovely way to bring the scent and positive effects of herbs and plants indoors. Hop pillows are traditionally associated with a good night's sleep and can easily be made by stuffing the hops into a small cushion cover, and re-covering with a pillow slip or similar. Keep this beside you when you lie in bed, and the relaxing effects should soon make insomnia a thing of the past.

Make smaller pockets full of lavender flowers or peppermint leaves to keep by your side or carry with you. These are wonderfully cooling for the warmer months, and crushing them gently will release a soothing and delightful aroma. Make similar pockets filled with rose petals and a few crushed cloves to have a warming and comforting effect, useful in the winter.

There are many household uses for plants and herbs, and pomanders, herb sachets and moth bags are especially useful. The simplest pomander can be made by taking a thick-skinned orange and piercing it all over with dried cloves. Tie a simple ribbon around it and hang wherever you need its spicy scent. Herb and flower sachets can continue the therapeutic effects of any remedy you are taking, by carrying the scent into your home. These simple pockets of dried material can be inserted into clothing drawers, tied to bedposts, and even placed between sheets of writing paper to make sure that the scent permeates every area of your life. Choose from the deliciously-scented range of lavender, violet, rosemary, rose, basil, anise, and any other that you truly enjoy.

Many dried herbs are effective moth repellents and can be scattered over clothes and linen that is not in frequent use. Make a small pocket out of cotton fabric, and pack with southernwood, woodruff, rosemary, mint, thyme, sage, sweet marjoram, lavender and mugwort. Add a pinch of crushed cloves to round out the scent, and hang in the wardrobe, attach to hangers, and use wherever moths can be a problem.

REVIEW OF AILMENTS

Common Ailments
These are guidelines. If symptoms persist or recur regularly, consult your

Health Concern	Dietary Measure	Treatment Choice
Aches and Pains	Increase fresh fruit and vegetables and consider a juice fast	Dissolve 1 lb Epsom Salts in a hot bath and soak
Arthritis	Avoid coffee, wine, pepper, animal protein and wheat	Regular heat wraps and apply ginger compress to the liver. Express feelings and emotions regularly through any creative medium
Athlete's Foot	Reduce sugar, yeast and wheat, and limit mushrooms	Cover with honey and leave on overnight
Back Pain	Fast for pain relief and then bowel cleanse to ease congestion	Assume the Osteopathic Rescue Position and apply ice pack
Bad Breath	Overhaul diet and instigate regular fruit and juice fasts	Chew a small bunch of fresh parsley after meals, or fennel, cardamom or caraway seeds

natural healthcare practitioner for specific personalised advice.

Natural Remedy	Prevention	Page
Take Mag. Phos. tissue salt until relieved	Keep eliminative channels open — ensure good bowel health by skin brushing and drink plenty of water	79, 134, 148, 184, 200
Supplement with Glucosamine Sulphate and Vitamin C daily to improve mobility and reduce pain	Exercise with good joint protection	57, 77, 203
Wash with dilute solution of Ti-Tree essential oil	Good foot hygiene and regular exercise. Pee on feet occasionally	177, 199
Apply warm compress with Crab Apple flower remedy	Practise good posture, lifting and movement, and have annual structural check-up	37, 91, 108, 172, 200
Skin brush to improve general elimination and drink plenty of water. Take 2 naturally activated charcoal tablets	Ensure good mouth and bowel health	79, 80, 148

Health Concern	Dietary Measure	Treatment Choice
Breathing difficulties	Reduce wheat and cow's dairy	Massage therapy on chest and spine
Bruising	Increase fresh foods and have regular fruit and vegetable fasts. Include lettuce, watercress and fresh coriander leaves in juices	Massage the area with dilute essential oil of thyme
Burns (minor)	Drink lots of fluids and see Shock below	Cool as quickly as possible, then spray with soluble Vitamin C and cover with honey
Colds	Fluid or juice fast. Add fresh thyme to cooking	Stay warm and get plenty of rest
Constipation	Increase fruit and vegetable fibre, and have warm, stewed figs, prunes or apple every day. Eat 1 teaspoon of ginger in a pot of live yoghurt	Instigate a programme of regular Sitz Baths and abdominal massage
Corns and bunions	Ensure adequate amounts of olive, sesame or sunflower oil in diet	Soak feet regularly in hot salt water and massage with warmed sesame oil

Natural Remedy	Prevention	Page
Steam inhalations with herbal decongestants	Regular deep-breathing exercise, and Tone or Chant	109, 114, 115, 135, 146, 148, 207
Supplement with Vitamin C and Rutin daily	Regular exercise and massage to improve circulation	57, 79, 109
Supplement with Vitamin C and Vitamin E every 4 hours on that day		57
Drink lemon juice sweetened with honey and topped with hot water	Take 10 drops of Echinacea tincture or extract daily for 3 weeks each month	23, 57, 79, 115, 201
Drink warmed prune juice before bed each night. Take fresh blackberry juice when available	Walk every day, especially on an incline. Develop lower abdominal muscles with careful and specific exercise	58, 98, 132
Paint corns with neat Ti-Tree essential oil	Postural assessment and well-fitting shoes. Exercise feet and toes regularly, and consider reflexology treatment	92, 109, 178

Health Concern	Dietary Measure	Treatment Choice
Cystitis	Eat plenty of asparagus and parsnips to strengthen the bladder. Drink plenty of good water every day	Sit in a warm bath and drink as much water and dilute cranberry juice as you can
Diarrhoea	Have warm, sweet drinks and small meals. Begin by having 1 dry matzo cracker with a glass of warm apple juice every 2 hours	Ensure plenty of rest, and once able, sip flat Coca-Cola
Earache	Sip warm clove tea. Take only liquids if pain is acute, otherwise add garlic, ginger and olive oil or ghee to the diet	Warm some sweet almond oil, soak a cotton wool ball in it and use to plug the ear. Cover for comfort and to hold the heat in
Eczema	Reduce wheat and dairy products, and increase rice (preferably basmati) and oats	Wash with oatmeal bags, not soap, and soak in an oatmeal bath each day

Natural Remedy	Prevention	Page
Add a strong Yarrow decoction or infusion to a hip bath and relax in it every day	Always add a capful of apple cider vinegar to bathwater, ensure excellent toilet habits (always wipe from front to back) and sexual protocol — always pee as soon as decently possible after intercourse.	134, 167
Supplement with Acidophilus and Bifidus once normal diet is resumed	Avoid antibiotics, ensure good food choices and hygiene, minimise animal proteins and never eat your emotions and feelings!	60
Gargle with warm dilute lemon juice and supplement with Vitamin C	Avoid draughts, check health of tonsils/adenoids and consider cranial therapy	57, 200
Supplement with zinc and EFA for 3 weeks each month	Identify and treat food and contact allergies — use a diet diary and consider elimination and cleansing diets	56, 63

Health Concern	Dietary Measure	Treatment Choice
Gas	Reduce beans and fried foods and cook with a pinch of ginger spice and asafoetida	Take 2 naturally activated charcoal tablets
Gout	Restrict pepper, animal produce, alcohol and wheat	Juice fast regularly to rebalance the system
Hayfever	Eliminate cow's dairy produce and wheat. Limit cold foods and drinks, especially ices	Apply a fresh onion poultice to the back of the neck
Headaches	Follow a light diet and introduce regular grape fasts	Apply a warm compress to the back of the neck and lie down to relieve muscle tension
Indigestion	Monitor meal size and consider food combining. Have regular fruit and vegetable juice fasts, especially pineapple, apple and celery	Add digestive aids like dill herb, cooked onions and fresh mint to meals

Natural Remedy	Prevention	Page
Supplement with Acidophilus and Bifidus	Overhaul diet to identify individual food intolerance and introduce good alternatives. Consider food combining as a short-term measure	71, 72, 78
Eat black cherries with meals and drink the juice daily	Work on restoring acid/alkaline balance through dietary change and remedial fasts	56, 79
Take Nat. Mur. tissue salt and supplement with Vitamin C	Hum regularly to clear the nasal passages and sinuses. Smear nostrils with Vaseline or sesame oil to screen out pollen	57, 115, 184
Crush a handful of fresh lemon balm leaves, breathe deeply and apply to forehead	Identify and treat any food triggers. Get regular exercise and fresh air, and avoid draughts	79, 125, 201, 203, 207
Take camomile, fennel and peppermint teas as a digestive after meals	Eat in calm and restful situations, and consider all the influences on your digestion, including noise and other disturbances	52, 79, 164

Health Concern	Dietary Measure	Treatment Choice
Insect bites and stings	Eat lots of garlic every day	Apply neat Ti-Tree oil directly to each bite
Low energy.	Eat some carbohydrate every 3-4 hours, even if it is just a small snack. Follow a grape fast every month	Take Combination B tissue salt for a quick and effective energy lift
Migraines	Avoid cheese, fermented foods and chocolate. Add olive oil, grapefruit and pineapple juices to regular diet	Apply cool compress to forehead and back of neck and focus your attention on keeping hands cool, and then warming them again
Mouth ulcers and cold sores	Ensure daily fresh foods and juices	Squeeze drops from a fresh, organic lemon directly onto the sore 3-5 times a day
Nausea	Check for food allergies/intolerance. Limit caffeine and increase fluids. Drink lots of good water	Chew a small piece of crystallised ginger, or a small handful of fresh caraway seeds, and take a cup of warm camomile tea. Practise deep, relaxed breathing

Natural Remedy	Prevention	Page
Wash site of bee stings with a solution of bicarbonate of soda, and wasp stings with dilute vinegar	Wear or carry a handkerchief soaked in strong Pennyroyal tea, or a small posy of the fresh herb	178
Supplement with 30mg Coenzyme Q a day, and take Iron as a tissue salt or in liquid form (Floradix)	Ensure diet is rich in seaweed and sea vegetables. Have regular health checks, and get enough sleep, exercise and fresh air	58, 181
Take a cup of strong black coffee to avert an attack	Stress management, postural assessment, and regular expression of emotions, especially the more difficult ones such as anger and resentment	75, 207
Supplement with Vitamin C and sip 1 cup of licorice tea each day during an outbreak	Supplement with L-lysine and monitor amino-acid balance of diet. Also check integrity of dental fillings	57
Supplement with B-complex vitamins	Ensure good basic diet and maintain bowel health and regularity	145, 163

Health Concern	Dietary Measure	Treatment Choice
Period troubles	Follow a fruit or vegetable fast for 3 days at ovulation. Eat extra vegetable and fruit fibre, soya and miso to decongest the pelvis and regulate the cycle	Keep lower body warm — sandwich pelvis between hot water bottles and soak feet if necessary in warm water
Poor appetite	Ensure regular mealtimes and plenty of variety	Drink ginger tea 30 minutes before a meal
Prostate concerns	Add pumpkins, squashes, pumpkin seeds and asparagus to the diet. Eliminate animal fats	Take barley water drink spiced with clove and saffron
Shock	If there is no major injury, take sweet drink, or take or apply 5 drops of Rescue Remedy	Sit or lie on the ground, breathe deeply and fully, and then have a hot mustard footbath
Sinus complaints	Eliminate cow's dairy and ensure good alternatives. Have plenty of warm drinks	Apply a warm compress and take a steam inhalation with fresh rosemary or thyme

Natural Remedy	Prevention	Page
Take Mag. Phos. tissue salt for cramps	Consider a monthly retreat to revitalise and renew energy levels	37, 58, 59, 132, 134
Supplement with Iron as a tissue salt or in liquid form (Floradix). Use digestive spices such as fennel, caraway, cumin and ginger with meals	At least once each week, take fenugreek tea sweetened with molasses	52
Supplement with Saw Palmetto berries	Ensure regular health checks	165
Wash your surrounding area with a dilution of lemongrass essential oil	Stay alert and don't sleepwalk through your life	153
Sip several cups of black pepper tea and massage the face and neck with an oil blend to which black pepper essential oil has been added	Regularly treat skin to a salt glow or scrub to help elimination through the skin	79, 115, 175, 201

Health Concern	Dietary Measure	Treatment Choice
Sleeplessness	Take a warm, milky drink before bed	Sip alternately 1 cup of strong black coffee, and 1 of camomille tea
Sprains and Strains	Check any overweight, and ensure adequate protein in the diet	Rest the area then apply ice, then light pressure, and raise the affected part above the level of your heart
Sunburn	Liquid-only diet until fully recovered	Wash area with vinegar diluted in tepid water, and apply cool yoghurt
Thrush	Eliminate yeast and sugar, and eat plenty of live yoghurt	Apply fresh, live yoghurt to cool and soothe, and bathe the area with well-diluted apple cider vinegar
Warts	Cleanse and tone the blood with salad leaves, bitter herbs and nettles	Apply neat organic lemon juice and expose to the sun 3 times a day

Natural Remedy	Prevention	Page
Lie on a hop pillow or place 2 drops of Clary Sage essential oil on the pillow slip	Expend energy during the day, practise relaxation, manage stress, and leave worries and anxieties outside the bedroom	177
Supplement with 1g Vitamin C every 3 hours while the pain persists, and take Vitamin C and Dolomite regularly	Ensure good muscle tone and exercise habits, e.g. always wear the right clothes and supports, and warm up properly	57, 99, 129–30
Supplement with Vitamin C, bioflavonoids and Vitamin E	Always protect your skin	57, 198
Supplement with 1g Vitamin C and Echinacea tincture or extract daily	Let the area breathe. Take B-complex Vitamins and Acidopholus with Bifidus after any course of antibiotics	57, 197
Take Thuja extract or tincture daily for 3 weeks	Pep up the immune system with Echinacea and Vitamin C for 3 weeks out of every month	54, 57

RESOURCES

A Natural Medicine Chest

Access to fresh water and the elements of the natural world often provide an answer to minor first-aid needs. A range of herbs, flowers and natural ingredients can form the basis of a personal medicine chest that will meet your needs and those of your family. Beyond any home-made remedies such as tinctures, infusions and syrups, you may like to buy in some of the following cures to ensure you have a naturally-based answer to all your immediate healthcare needs. These are the cures I use most often, and you can tailor your own medicine chest to meet your individual needs and those of your family.

- Dr Bach Rescue Remedy and Rescue Cream — instant relief from all manner of ills
- Ti-Tree and Lemongrass Essential Oils — powerful antiseptic and disinfectants
- Arnica cream and tablets — for all injuries, bruising and shock
- Calendula cream — to treat all skin complaints
- Echinacea tincture — an immediate boost for the immune system
- Nat. Mur. and Mag. Phos. Tissue Salts — choose your own constitutional remedies, or those which cover the most common incidents in your life
- Peppermint and Licorice Root teas — to treat all manner of stomach and digestive concerns
- Vitamin C and Vitamin E capsules — for internal and external use.

Finding a Practitioner

Your health is one of your greatest assets, and it is an area where you are the specialist. Any health adviser or healthcare practitioner that you work with will need to respect and augment your wisdom, finding ways to interpret your own unique recipe for full health *with* you, and providing information and support for how best to get the most from your individual resources.

Choose a practitioner with whom you can get along; you want to be able to discuss everything and anything with this person. Also look for somebody trustworthy who inspires you. These qualities are invaluable in terms of the relationship that you will build between you. Look also to the practitioner's own health and stress levels, to see how successful he or she is in meeting personal health and lifestyle challenges.

Enquire about any aspects of the practitioner's work that seem especially relevant or of interest to you, and any particular sphere of influence or specialty and experience. Professional associations will hold registers of practitioners who have completed their training courses, and this is a good place to begin when looking for a practitioner. Ask around, too, because personal recommendation is a real reference. Check with your friends, and also with your local healthfood shop manager, pharmacist and GP. Sometimes experienced practitioners will not be members of their professional Associations for reasons of politics or whatever. The world of Natural Medicine is going through a process of immense change as professional bodies are becoming more organised and uniform, and this will be a positive move when things are finalised, resulting in a more streamlined and professional approach throughout. In the meantime, it can be difficult for the public to access the practitioners that they need, so persevere in your search for a practitioner with whom you can work successfully.

Practitioners all work in different ways and will use a synthesis of their own personal skills and whatever professional training they may have undertaken. Generally, a naturopath, nature cure practitioner or natural healthcare practitioner will be able to fulfil a total GP-type function, embracing a wealth of different healthcare measures that will all serve to enhance your own health and well-being. They will generally be able to address all your health concerns, and may refer you on to other specialist practitioners. They will all use a slightly different blend of techniques and approaches, depending upon their own strengths and preferences, but you should find that the three main arms of healthcare are covered:

- Structural health — either through the use of osteopathy or a gentler technique
- System health — through diet and lifestyle advice
- Mental/Emotional health — through counselling and awareness techniques

The emphasis throughout will be on educating you to work for yourself to improve your own healthcare.

There is an enormous variety of natural therapies available to Nature Cure practitioners. They may be employed by your main healthcare advisor, or you may be referred to another practitioner for these. The following is a selection of useful health-enhancing specialties which all come under the umbrella of Nature Cure.

- Aromatherapy
- Affirmations
- Analysis
- Body work, e.g. Bioenergetics

- Clay therapy
- Counselling
- Cranial work
- Creative therapies
- Detoxification
- Energy work, e.g. Shiatsu
- Healing
- Kinesiology
- Meditation
- Naturopathic Dietary Therapy
- Osteopathy
- Relaxation and Stress Management
- Reflexology
- Spiritual guidance and practices
- Therapeutic Massage

Methods of Diagnosis

When you consult a naturopath or nature cure practitioner, he or she will use a number of different techniques to ascertain the fullest possible picture of your health. Each initial visit will last anywhere between one and two hours; this is to allow the fullest possible time for the taking of your medical and personal health history, and to make a full diagnosis of your current state of health. Treatment or advice will also be included based on the findings of investigations and the conclusions that you reach about how best to work together.

Practitioners will reach their conclusions about your current health in consultation with you, and through a variety of different ways, some of which may be new to you. Occasionally blood and other tests will be taken, but in the main these diagnostic tools are non-invasive.

They may include:

- Facial and Tongue Diagnosis — achieved by looking closely at your features and the markings on your tongue.
- Structural Assessment — a full physical examination of the structure and function of your body, and how and where your feelings manifest themselves.
- Iridology or Iris Diagnosis — close study of the iris using a gentle light and a magnifying glass; photographs may be taken.
- Neurological Testing — examination of the nervous system through structural integrity using gentle movement and stimulus.
- Applied Kinesiology (Muscle Response Testing) — a comprehensive system of testing the responsiveness of major muscle groups and individual areas and sites in the body.
- Allergy testing — using safe exposure to suspected allergens.

The practitioner will also test your responsiveness to particular remedies and ways of working, and will look for any affinity with different treatment options. He or she will also observe your general ease of movement, your ability to relax and your capacity to utilise other skills such as visualisations.

Professional Associations

Institute for Complementary Medicine
15 Tavern Quay, London SE16 1QZ. Tel: 1071 237 5165

Irish Association of Holistic Medicine
9–11 Grafton Street, Dublin 2. Tel: (353) 1 671 2788

Incorporated Society of British Naturopaths
Kingston, The Coach House, 293 Gilmerton Road, Edinburgh EH16 5UQ. Tel: 0131 664 3435

Suppliers and other Useful Addresses

NUTRITIONAL AIDS

Lamberts Nutritional Supplies
1 Lamberts Road, Tunbridge Wells, Kent TN2 3EQ. Tel: 01892 552121

FSC Quality Vitamins
Europa Park, Stoneclough Road, Radcliffe, Manchester M26 1GG. Tel: 01204 707420

Sona Nutrition Ltd
IDA Business Centre, IDA Industrial Park, Whiteheaven, Dublin 24. Tel: (353) 1 4515087

ESSENTIAL OILS

Fragrant Earth
PO Box 182, Taunton, Somerset TA1 1SD. Tel: 01823 335734

Verde Essential Oils
75 Northcote Road, Battersea, London SW11. Tel: 0171 924 4379

Herbs

Potters Herbal Suppliers
Leyland Mill Lane, Wigan WN1 2SB. Tel: 01942 34761

Chi Dynamics

Gaye Wright
Creative Life Company, PO Box 227, Lutwyche, Queensland 4030, Australia.

General

Compassion in World Farming
20 Lavant Street, Petersfield, Hants GU32 3EW.

The Soil Association
86–88 Colston Street, Bristol, Avon BS1 5BB.

The Herb Society
PO Box 599, London SW11 4RW.

Recommended Further Reading

Chapter 1 Introduction

Adams, Richard and Max Hooper, *Nature through the Seasons*, Penguin 1975
Roet, Stephen, *All in the Mind*, Optima 1989
Storm, Hyemehosts, *Seven Arrows*, Ballantine 1984

Chapter 2 Individual Health

Chopra, Deepak, *Perfect Health*, Bantam 1990
Hartvig, Kirsten and Dr Nic Rowley, *Your Are What You Eat*, Piatkus 1996
Hope-Murray, Angela and Tony Pickup, *Healing with Ayurveda*, Newleaf 1997
Meadows, Kenneth, *Earth Medicine*, Element 1989
Viagas, Belinda Grant, *A–Z of Natural Healthcare*, Newleaf 1997

Chapter 3 Food and Drink

Bartimeus, Paula, *Eating with the Seasons*, Element 1997
Cowmeadow, Oliver and Michele Cowmeadow, *Yin-Yang Cookbook*, Optima 1988
Grant, Belinda, *Detox Diet Book*, Optima 1991
Hartvig, Kirsten and Dr Nic Rowley, *You Are What You Eat*, Piatkus 1996
Mascetti, Manuela Dunn and Arunima Borthwick, *Food for the Soul*, Newleaf 1997
Singha, Shyam, *The Secrets of Natural Health*, Element 1997

Chapter 4 Energy, Movement and Healing

Balcombe, Betty, *As I See It*, Piatkus 1988
Meadows, Kenneth, *The Medicine Way*, Element 1990
Ohasi, Waturo, *Do-it-Yourself Shiatsu*, Japan Publications Inc.
Portugues, Gladys and Joyce Vedral, *Hard Bodies*, Thorsons 1986
Sneddon, Peta and Paolo Coseschi, *Healing with Osteopathy*, Newleaf 1996

Chapter 5 The Elements

Burgess, Jacquie, *Healing with Crystals*, Newleaf 1997
Meadows, Kenneth, *Shamanic Experience*, Element 1991
Viagas, Belinda Grant, *Natural Healthcare for Women*, Newleaf 1997

Chapter 6 Nature's Gifts

Culpepper, Nicholas, *Culpepper's Complete Herbal*, W. Foulsham and Co. Ltd
Harvey, Clare G. and Amanda Cochrane, *The Encyclopaedia of Flower Remedies*, Thorsons 1994
Hoad, Judith, *Healing with Herbs*, Newleaf 1996
Lawless, Julia, *The Illustrated Encyclopedia of Essential Oils*, Element 1995
Mindell, Earl, *The Vitamin Bible*, Arlington Books
Stanway, Dr Andrew, *A Guide to Biochemic Tissue Salts*, Van Dyke Books

Chapter 7 The Kitchen Pharmacy

Campion, Kitty, *Kitty Campion's Handbook of Herbal Health*, Sphere 1985
Morningstar, Amadea with Urmila Desai, *The Ayurvedic Cookbook*, Lotus Press 1990
Treben, Maria, *Health from God's Garden*, Thorsons 1987
Viagas, Belinda Grant, *Natural Remedies for Common Complaints*, Piatkus 1995

General Titles

Balcombe, Betty, *The Energy Connection*, Piatkus 1993
Illych, Ivan, *Medical Nemesis*, Pelican 1977
Meadows, Kenneth, *Where Eagles Fly*, Element 1995
Oxenford, Rosalind, *Healing with Reflexology*, Newleaf 1996
Sams, Jamie, *The 13 Original Clan Mothers*, Harper Collins 1993
Schaef, Anne Wilson, *When Society becomes an Addict*, Permanent Publications 1987
Trattler, Ross, ND DO, *Better Health through Natural Healing*, Thorsons 1985
Zeuss, Jonathan, *The Wisdom of Depression*, Newleaf 1999

Further Information

To contact the author, for news of trainings and workshops, and for details of her postal Advice Service, please write to:

Belinda Grant Viagas PO Box 13386, London NW3 2ZE